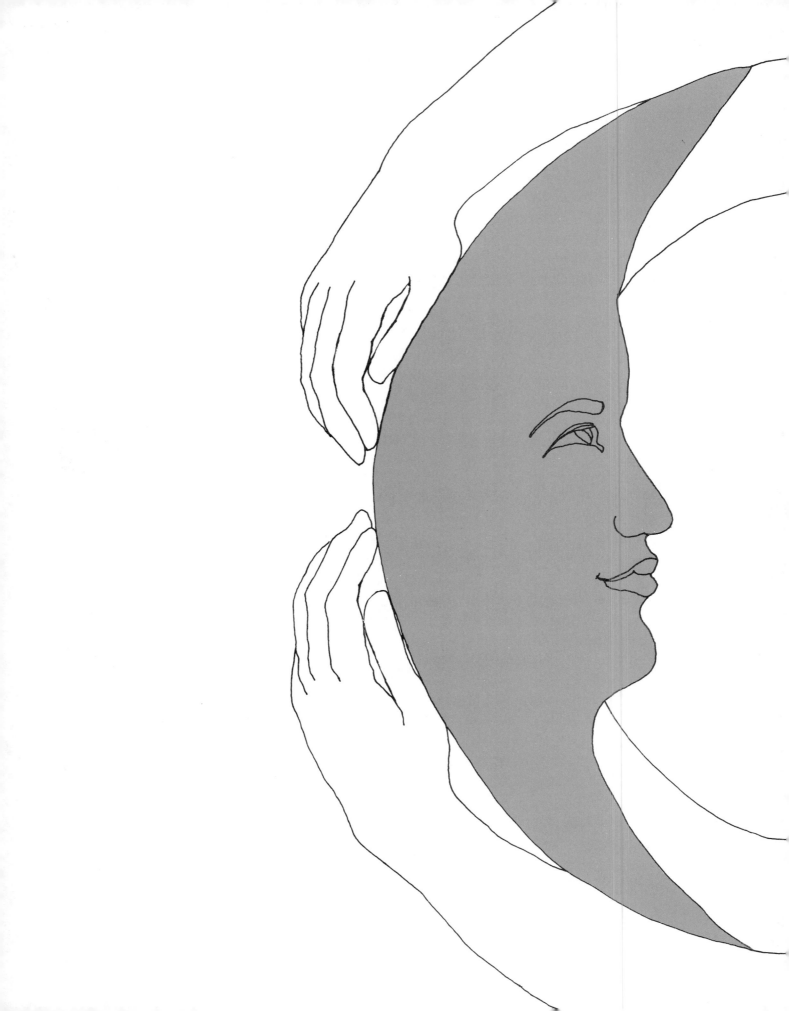

THE
MASSAGE
BOOK

GEORGE DOWNING

ILLUSTRATED BY
ANNE KENT RUSH

RANDOM HOUSE - THE BOOKWORKS

This work was originally published in slightly different form in 1972 by Random House, Inc.

The illustrator wishes to acknowledge the use of copyright material from
Art Students' Anatomy by Edmond J. Farris, Dover Publications, Inc., New York
(which appears on the following pages: 169 through 179);
reprinted through permission of the publisher.

Photo page 182 by John Pearson

This book is co-published by Random House, Inc., 201 East 50th Street, New York,
New York 10022, and The Bookworks, Berkeley, California

Cover design, book design: Anne Kent Rush
Typesetting by Vera Allen Composition Service, Hayward, California

ISBN 0-679-77789-X

Random House website address: www.atrandom.com

Printed in the United States of America on acid-free paper

24689753

Twenty-fifth Anniversary Edition

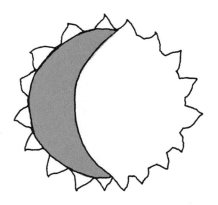

CONTENTS

CONTENTS

LET THERE BE BACK RUBS!

Until the January 1972 publication of *The Massage Book,* massage in the United States was practiced only by medical therapists, sex-parlor workers, and professional trainers. *The Massage Book* changed that by making available to the general public little-known techniques for muscle relaxation and healing touch. In a brief time, massage went from being an obscure profession to a pleasurable part of most people's everyday lives.

The Massage Book has been voted one of the three "most influential books of the past twenty-five years" by *Natural Health* magazine (March–April 1996), and the reason behind this becomes clear when we try to imagine life without massage. Imagine that there are no books on massage in bookstores; health clubs have no masseurs; massage oil is not on sale anywhere; spas don't offer massage to tired vacationers. Back rub stores don't dot the avenues of large cities. Doctors and insurance companies don't consider massage as therapy after accidents. You'd like to help an ailing child or parent or friend feel better, but you don't know how. On a romantic weekend, your lover doesn't include a sensual massage among the menu of treats. Surely, life before massage was much less comfortable.

In 1970, after I moved from Boston to Berkeley, the idea for this book came to me during my first encounter with California body therapies. I worked in publishing, and a manual on massage for the layperson seemed like a delicious, helpful idea. Later, when I joined the teaching staff at Esalen Institute, I suggested this idea to my colleague George Downing. We agreed that he would write the book and I would illustrate it. The Bookworks in Berkeley had the vision to publish it, and Random House agreed to copublish. Downing and I recruited our neighbors—and even our editor, Don Gerrard, and his wife, Eugenia—as models for my illustrations. After publication, we smiled our way through a promotional tour in which many talk-show hosts sniggered nervously at the topic. But the public embraced massage wholeheartedly, and our book became a huge bestseller.

The Massage Book has been in print for more than twenty-five years and has become a classic, essential manual for learning massage. I have gone on to write ten more books on different kinds of body therapies, but this book is still one of my favorites. This Twenty-fifth Anniversary Edition is a celebration of the pleasures *The Massage Book* has brought us by broadening our vision and providing us with the permission to touch each other in a relaxed, caring way. I hope this book becomes one of your favorites too. Give, receive, and enjoy!

—Anne Kent Rush
Telluride, Colorado, 1998

WHY MASSAGE

Massage is for your mate, your family, and your friends. It is for grandmothers and babies, for pets, for those you love and, if you are up to it, for those you hate. To do massage is physically to help someone, to take care of them. It is for anyone with whom you feel prepared to share an act of physical caring.

Contrary to myth, massage is a healing art and not an advanced sexual technique. Naturally, when practiced by lovers, it can be a beautiful extension of sexuality. The flowing peace and aliveness it so easily brings to the body can be channeled, if both parties desire things so, in that direction. But this is merely one of the many possibilities that massage holds out to us.

The core of massage lies in its unique way of communicating without words. In itself this is not unusual; by touching and hugging, for example, we often let those around us know that we like them, or that we sympathize with them, or that we believe in their worth. Massage, however, can transpose this kind of message into a new and different key. When receiving a good massage a person usually falls into a mental-physical state difficult to describe. It is like entering a special room until now locked and hidden away; a room the very existence of which is likely to be familiar only to those who practice some form of daily meditation. By itself this state is a gift. However, he who is giving the massage need not stop there. The more he can tune in to his friend's heightened awareness, the more he can convey something of his own inner self and experience as well. The least touch becomes a statement, like drawing with a fine pen on sensitive paper. Trust, empathy and respect, to say nothing of a sheer sense of mutual physical existence, for this moment can be expressed with a fullness never matched by words.

In its essence massage is something simple. It makes us more whole, more fully ourselves. Your hands have the power to give this to others. Learn to trust that power and you will quickly find out better than anyone can tell you what massage is all about.

HOW TO USE THIS BOOK

I have written this book with two ends in mind: to tell you how to do massage, and to explain a little of what I see as its meaning and purpose.

The first third of the book contains a lot of practical information which you will want to know before you begin: the nature of massage oils, how to do massage on the floor as opposed to doing it on a massage table and the like. If you have never done massage before, I strongly suggest that you read through these chapters before tackling the later parts of the book. In particular take a good look at "How to Use Your Hands." Even if you already know some massage I would recommend at least a glance at this chapter.

In the middle third of the book you will find instructions on how to give, stroke by stroke and body part by body part, a long and thorough complete massage. The type described is one of many possible variations of what has come to be known as Esalen-style massage. This approach to massage, developed in recent years at Esalen Institute in Big Sur and San Francisco, is in turn a variation of a European tradition over a century old, commonly called Swedish massage. Many of the techniques I teach in my own workshops for Esalen are included in this section.

The type, the illustrations, and the physical design of this book have been planned in order to make it as convenient as possible for you to have it open at your side when you want to try doing some massage with a friend. However, before you start be sure to read over both the short introduction to the instruction section and the particular descriptions of whatever strokes you wish to try out. I would also advise you to start small; don't try to learn more than a half dozen strokes or so at one sitting. Finally, whenever you get a chance, have the strokes you are attempting to learn done to you as well.

Don't worry, incidentally, if as you thumb through this book the strokes in the instruction section look difficult to you. In actual practice they are much easier than they look to be on paper. Numerous people who originally knew no massage have tested portions of this book before it was printed. All found little difficulty in learning the strokes once they actually tried them.

The final third of the book is designed to help you develop your own personal massage style. To this end I have included a series of more advanced technical suggestions, some brief information about other types and traditions of massage, and, most important, some comments about the meaning of massage and how an understanding of this meaning can aid you in doing better work with your hands. Read this part of the book whenever you like, but I suspect that it won't make a great deal of sense until you have become fairly familiar with the material presented in the instruction section. Master a few basic techniques first. Then, with a glance at a few of the guideposts in the last part of this book, by all means go on from there.

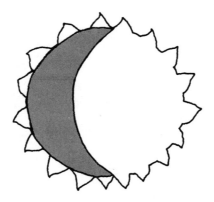

OILS AND POWDERS

The only really good way to do massage is with oil. Your hands cannot apply pressure and at the same time move smoothly over the surface of the skin without some kind of lubricating agent. Oil fulfills this function better than anything else.

The two kinds of oil most commonly used for massage are vegetable oil and mineral oil. As far as lubrication goes they are equally satisfactory. Mineral oil is used in almost all professional studios because it is the cheaper of the two. My own preference, however, is very much for vegetable oil.

My reasons, I admit, are based largely upon intuition and hearsay. Ever since the widespread realization that natural foods are more healthful for us there has arisen a massive underground lore concerning, among other things, the care and treatment of the skin; one especially frequent claim is that vegetable oil is good for your skin and mineral oil is bad for it. Why? Well, answers one person, vegetable oil is easily absorbed by the skin whereas mineral oil tends to clog the pores. And, responds another, vegetable oil adds vitamins to the skin whereas mineral oil if anything destroys certain ones. And so forth. Whether any or all such reasons are true, I don't really know; nor, so far, have I come across any solid scientific research pointing one way or the other. Yet my own bones seem to vibrate with the same general message, and until I see proof to the contrary I intend to keep on massaging and getting massaged with vegetable oil.

Given that you are using a vegetable oil, what particular vegetable it happens to come from does not, I suspect, greatly matter. Everyone does seem to have his own favorite; at the moment I find myself in an almond oil phase. In the past, however, I have used olive oil, safflower oil, avocado oil and numerous others; and all with equal satisfaction. Safflower oil, which is certainly as good as any of the others, has the advantage of being relatively inexpensive, and both safflower oil and olive oil have the further advantage of being available at almost any grocery store. Most other vegetable oils you can find on the shelves of a good health food store. All of them, incidentally, can be mixed in any combination with other oils.

Baby oil? If this is all you have around you can get by with it. It is quite difficult to use, however, because it soaks so quickly into the skin that during a massage new applications become necessary every few minutes. Hand lotions are even less satisfactory for the same reason.

Whatever oil you use, mineral, vegetable or other, it is more than likely to be neutral or worse in odor. If so, be sure to add something to it that will give it a pleasant scent. Musk is one of my own favorites; several drops added to a cup of oil will usually do nicely. Concentrated clove oil, cinnamon oil, and lemon oil work well and can be bought at some drugstores. Today many head shops carry a wide variety of imported scented oils. Frangipani, a concentrated oil imported from India, is an especially popular one.

Once I even found a concentrated chocolate oil. This didn't work out so well, as I kept getting hungry in the middle of the massage.

A nice idea is to keep a variety of mixed oils with different scents on hand, and then to let whomever you massage choose the one he or she prefers. Picking a favorite oil usually makes a person a little more immediately receptive to being massaged with it.

Keep your oils, once mixed and scented, in plastic bottles that are not easily upset and that have narrow openings, i.e., an eighth of an inch or smaller. Any store that has cosmetic supplies is a good place to look for bottles of this kind. Many shampoos and hand lotions also come in them.

What about powders? Well, they work. Not as well as oils do: you have to apply them more often, and they don't cut down the friction between your hands and your friend's skin nearly as effectively. But there may be times when you will want to use a powder. Like when you want to massage a friend who can't stand the feel of oil against his or her skin (it happens). Or when you have run out of oil. Or just for a change.

Any talcum powder will do. Use it just as you would an oil.

And what about using nothing at all, besides your own hands? Of course you can do this. But it makes a decent massage much more difficult to give. Most of the strokes that will be described in this book can't be done without oil or powder. A few can, however, as you will see. You can always do massage, no matter what is or isn't lying around to do it with.

In the meantime lay in a good stock of oils and powders.

WORKING ON THE FLOOR

The easiest way to do massage is on a massage table. But don't worry — if you don't have a table you can give a great massage working on the floor. It's a little more trouble and a little more tiring. Go about it in the right way, however, and you can cut these hassles to a minimum.

First, though, let me warn you about beds. Sleep on beds, do whatever else you want on beds, but don't try to do serious massage on them. The reason is that they are too soft to provide the kind of underlying support you need when you want to apply pressure. Try to press hard on someone lying on a bed and the only thing that happens is that he disappears into the mattress. Water beds are an exception because of their firm and exactly fitted support. Ordinarily, however, a bed is the worst possible place you could choose for giving a massage. Either get a table, or find ways to make yourself comfortable on the floor.

The main thing when working on the floor is to make sure that you have sufficient padding. A foam pad one or two inches thick works well. However, it ought to be both longer and wider than the amount of space that actually will be occupied by your friend: it should be 7' x 4' or even bigger. The reason for this is that you, who are to give the massage, will also need padding. Some strokes, for example, will require you to kneel next to your friend, and if you don't have something under your knees at these times you will end up needing a massage much more than your friend ever did.

If you have a foam pad too short or narrow to sit or kneel on beside your friend, then try to supplement it with whatever additional padding you can find.

Two or three sleeping bags can also be used. Even some thick blankets will help. Unzip the sleeping bags and spread them out to double width. Then pile up whatever bags and/or blankets you are using as shown in the illustration.

A single mattress taken from a bed and placed directly on the floor will also work,

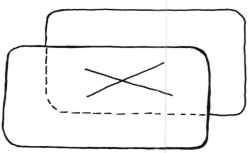

although its height from the floor makes it rather inconvenient to use. The thinner the mattress, the better.

Whatever padding you are using — foam, sleeping bags, blankets or whatever — cover it with a clean sheet before your friend lies down on it for his or her massage.

One minor problem that arises when working on the floor is that sooner or later you are going to knock over an oil bottle and spill some oil. If you are using a bottle with a sufficiently narrow opening, the amount of oil that will actually seep out will be very little. All the same, you may wish to take precautions against staining your rug, your sleeping bag, etc. The best preventive measure I have found is to purchase a large durable plastic sheet at a hardware store. Put the plastic sheet on top of whatever you want to protect, and then a bed sheet on top of the whole works. Also, the first time you use the plastic sheet take some tape and make an 'X' on the side that is up. Then when you fold the sheet to put it away make sure the "up" side gets folded against itself without ever coming into contact with the opposite side. This will keep you from someday putting the oily side of the sheet down on top of whatever you are trying to protect.

The actual massage techniques used while working on the floor differ very little from those used while working on a table. Where some specific stroke needs to be done in a different way I will mention it in the instruction section. However, I will add here two pieces of advice of a more general nature. One is always to give a somewhat shorter massage when working on the floor than you might if you were working on a table. This will keep you from getting tired out. The other is to bend your own back as little as possible while giving a massage. What this really means is, pay attention to where and how you are sitting or kneeling, taking every care to provide for your own comfort the whole while. That way you will give your friend a better massage, and will yourself enjoy giving it infinitely more.

A last remark. Nothing so enhances massage done on the floor as a fire in a nearby fireplace.

TABLES

Why a table? Its most important advantage is that it eliminates some bending and stooping as you work. This means that if you are giving a long massage your own back is less likely to get tired. A table also makes it easy for you to change your position with respect to the person you are massaging — from head to leg, from one side to the other side, etc. — without a break in the flow of your massage. Finally, it puts certain body parts (the sole of the foot, for example) more directly within the reach of your hands.

If you find that you are beginning to do a lot of massage, sooner or later you will probably want a table. In this case your options are three. You may find that some table which you already have around will, with perhaps a few modifications, serve well enough. Or you can buy one. Or you can build one.

The first requirement of a table is, naturally, that it be big enough that whomever you are going to massage can lie down on it, and sturdy enough to keep him or her there. Ideally the length and width should be about the same as that of your friend's body when he is lying flat with his arms close alongside his body; a professional massage table is usually six feet long and two feet wide, for example. However, if the only table you have available is either much too long or, as is more likely, much too wide, you can make do with it. What this means is that instead of just lying in one place while you do all the moving around, your friend will have to shift his or her position from time to time during a massage. A disadvantage, but hardly a disaster.

Height is equally important. Too low, and you will have to stoop; too high, and you won't get the leverage you need. Traditional massage lore gives two measures for the right height of a table. One is that it should be roughly as high from the floor as the top of your thighs. The other is that if you stand straight with your shoulders level you should be able to extend one arm straight down with the hand at a right angle (i.e., so that the hand is parallel to the floor), and have the palm of your hand just graze the surface of the table. Of these two measures I find the second more accurate, and find more accurate still the simple test of trying out the table by doing a little massage. For a man or woman of average size, 29 to 31 inches (including padding) is the right height range.

Sturdiness must also be considered. A table should be sturdy enough not only that your friend stays in place on it, but also that he or she doesn't worry about staying in place on it. If a table shakes and creaks with every stroke you can't very well expect your friend to relax on it.

Whatever the size and shape of the table you use, you must place some kind of padding on top for your friend to lie on. A one-inch foam pad is best. A sleeping bag will also work. The idea is to use something thick enough that whomever you massage will feel comfortable, yet thin enough that he or she won't bounce up and down under the varying pressure of your hands.

If you can't find a table that comes somewhat close to meeting these requirements, then the next step is either to build or to buy. Building a table can be fairly easy or fairly difficult, depending on how good you are with tools and how elaborate a table you decide to make.

The simplest and cheapest way to build your own massage table is to make two small sawhorses 28 inches or so high and 24 inches wide. (Any carpenter can also build them for you at little cost.) Then buy a piece of ¾ inch plywood cut 2 feet x 6 feet and a foam pad to match, and you are in business.

If you want to try something more elaborate, a friend of mine recently made a superb table that is both sturdy and easy to move and to store; it folds up into a neat package about 2 feet x 3 feet x 5 inches. Here is how you can build one too.

First assemble these materials:

— *2* sheets of ½ inch plywood 24 x 36 inches
— *3* sheets of ½ inch plywood 22 x 12 inches
— *4*-1 x 4 inch pine or fir boards 36 inches long
— *4*-1 x 4 inch pine or fir boards 22½ inches long
— *6*-2 x 2 inch boards 29 inches long
— *1*-24 inch continuous hinge
— *6* Stanley locking table leg braces #446¼ (be sure also to get instructions on how to place them)
— *2* handles
— *6*-3 inch strap hinges and screws
— *2* suitcase latches
— *8* brass corners

— nails (1½ inch finishing nails without heads are best. Bigger nails will split the wood.)

— a strong glue

(Note: these dimensions are for a table that will stand 30½ inches high including a one inch foam pad on top. If you want your table either higher or lower, just vary the length of the six 2 x 2 inch legs accordingly.)

Then construct the table as follows:

(1)   Cut the plywood and the boards for the frame and legs to size.

(2)   Build the frames, gluing and nailing the corners. (Make rabbit joints if you feel ambitious.)

(3)   Attach the tops and frames, gluing and nailing them. (If you still feel ambitious you can also "set in" the top.)

(4)   Hinge the legs to the undersides of the tops, gluing and nailing the crossbraces.

(5)   Attach the brackets. This is a tricky business, so try to follow the directions that come with them as closely as you can. You will have to play with them a little to find the exact placement spot.

(6)   Hinge the two halves of the table together.

(7)   Attach the catches, handles and corners.

(8)   Stain or varnish.

Put a one inch foam pad loose on top when you use the table.

If you want to buy a table there are some excellent ones on the market. Their chief advantage is that they are lightweight and portable: most of them are made of aluminum covered on the outside with either leather or naugahyde, and can be folded up into what looks like an overgrown attache case. Their chief drawback is their price, usually in the neighborhood of ninety to a hundred dollars. The best place to find or order one is at a large medical supplies house. Be sure to check out the measurements first, as some commercial portable tables appear to have been designed for massaging midgets.

Whatever kind of table you use, put a clean sheet over it and its padding when you are actually about to give a massage. A white sheet on a narrow table has, incidentally, a definite set of psychological overtones; use a colored sheet instead and you will keep your friend from getting a funny feeling that he or she is stretched out on the operating table waiting for the surgeon. Even better, buy a large piece of brightly colored terrycloth at a fabrics store.

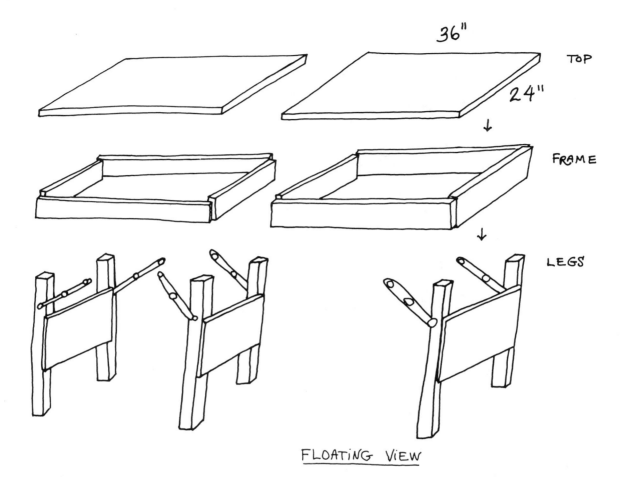

36"

24"

TOP

FRAME

LEGS

FLOATING VIEW

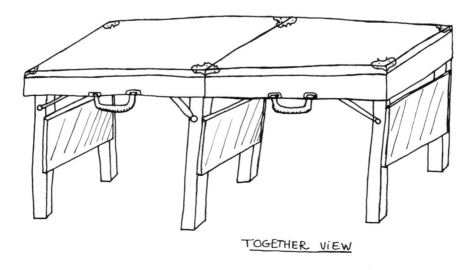

TOGETHER VIEW

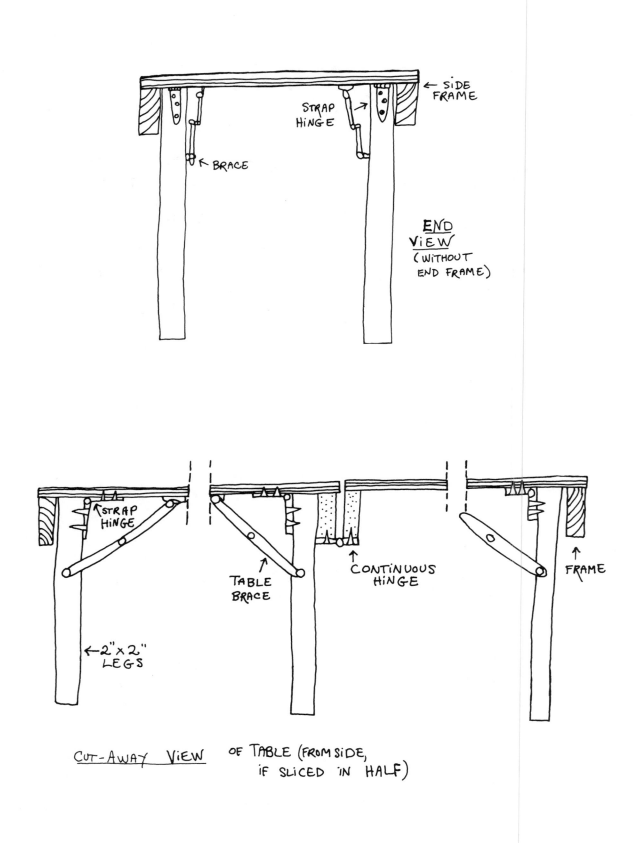

END
VIEW
(WITHOUT
END FRAME)

← SIDE
FRAME

STRAP
HINGE

← BRACE

STRAP
HINGE

TABLE
BRACE

CONTINUOUS
HINGE

FRAME

←2"×2"
LEGS

CUT-AWAY VIEW OF TABLE (FROM SIDE, IF SLICED IN HALF)

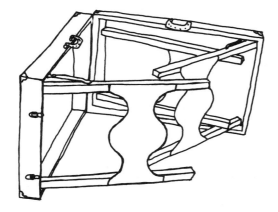

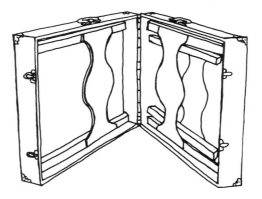

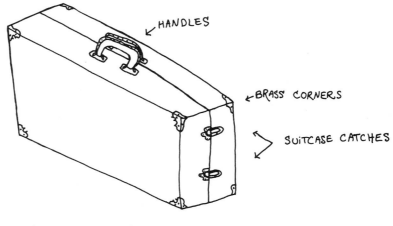

← HANDLES

← BRASS CORNERS

SUITCASE CATCHES

CLOSED TABLE

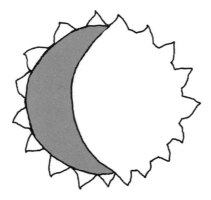

GETTING THINGS READY

Careful preparations and the right setting can make a good massage even better. Your friend will feel more comfortable, and you will too.

In choosing a place to give a massage the first thing to look for is solitude and quiet. A person receiving a massage enters a universe where the sense of touch alone is important; for this reason any outside noise and bustle can be extremely disconcerting.

The next thing to consider is warmth. Nothing destroys an otherwise good massage more quickly than physical coldness. The problem is the oil; a person with massage oil on his skin becomes easily chilled. The temperature in the room in which you give the massage should be about 70° or slightly over, and the room should be without drafts. Heat the room up before you begin; err, if in doubt, on the side of making it too warm. It is much easier to keep your friend feeling comfortable from the start than it is to warm him or her up once chilled.

For the same reason it is a good practice to keep a spare sheet on hand. Then, if during the massage your friend should begin to feel cold, you can use the sheet to cover the parts of his body you are not working on at the moment.

Make sure ahead of time that the oil is mixed and scented, that it is in a convenient container, that you have more than enough for a massage, and that it is warm. Warm means room temperature or close to it. If the oil is much cooler than this, warm it a little first before a fire or heater.

Arrange your table or your mat on the floor so that there is sufficient room for you to work on all four sides.

Don't use any kind of bright lighting that will fall directly on your friend's face. Even with his lids closed this will cause him to tense the muscles surrounding his eyes. In particular never use direct overhead lighting.

The question of music is a tricky one. Although I think that massaging to music can be a helpful exercise (how and why I will discuss in a later chapter), I strongly recommend that as a general rule you do not play music while giving a massage. I love music, don't get me wrong, and it certainly adds a pleasant relaxing atmosphere to a massage room, but I find at the same time that music tends to siphon off the deeper currents of a good massage experience. It is like trying to meditate to music: however beautiful it may be in itself, the music casts its own veil over everything you are feeling. On the other hand I must in all fairness admit that I know excellent masseurs and masseuses who like to both give and receive massages in this way. So I guess you will have to experiment and decide for yourself.

Check your own hands before giving a massage. The most important thing is to make sure your fingernails are short — the shorter, the better. I trim mine down as far as my scissors can reach before a massage.

Also wash your hands. Any grit or stickiness will make itself instantly felt.

And warm them if they are cold. Rub them briskly together for several minutes, or, if they are extremely cold, let them bask a little before a fire or heater.

If you have long hair tie it back so that it stays out of your eyes.

If you plan to stay dressed, wear loose clothing, so that you can move around easily; and dress as lightly as possible, since you will be working in a warm room. I might add that doing massage in the nude is extremely pleasant as long as no one on either side is uptight about it.

Both masseur or masseuse and massagee tend to get thirsty during a long massage, and a little water to drink can be a nice thing to have on hand. Even better, when the massage is over let your friend first rest for as long as he wishes with his eyes closed, and then when he opens his eyes offer him a glass of cold fruit juice.

Finally, if you ever have the chance to do massage outdoors, in the sun and surrounded by nature . . . need I say more?

WHAT TO TELL YOUR FRIEND

There are a few basic things one should know before receiving a massage. If you are the one who is going to give the massage, you will probably want to tell your friend something along the lines of the following comments.

The best way to receive a massage is in the nude. Even a minimal amount of clothing, e.g., underwear or a swimming suit, will get in the way of whoever is giving the massage, will require him or her to leave certain important muscle groups unmassaged, and will deny you what is perhaps the single most pleasant sensation of a complete massage, that of the total wholeness and connectedness of your body. If, however, to remove all your clothes would make you feel extremely nervous, then leave something on. The main thing, after all, is that you enjoy your massage. But do take off whatever you comfortably can.

Also remove rings, bracelets, necklaces, earrings, glasses and anything in your hair. And most important of all (so that your eyes can be massaged), contact lenses.

Whoever is giving you the massage will tell you whether first to lie down on your stomach or on your back. Either way, make sure that the top of your head is roughly even with the end of the table or the padding on which you are lying. Rest your arms at your sides.

Once you feel settled in place close your eyes. Then focus your attention on your breathing; this will almost immediately bring you more in touch with your entire body. Breathe either through the nose or the mouth. Let your breath get as long and smooth as it wants to be without, however, forcing it to do so, and let it flow as deep towards or into the pelvis as it can go. Try to sink yourself more and more into the present moment, letting thoughts drift out of your mind as easily as they have drifted in.

From this point on your job is simply to let yourself be completely taken care of. Don't try to "help" with the massage in any way. When it is time for your arm to be lifted, let it be lifted for you. When your head has to be turned to one side, let the turning be done by your friend. I repeat: don't try to "help" in any way; this can only cause a break in the relaxing flow of the massage. Instead keep your body as limp as you can manage, so that even when a limb is being lifted it would fall instantly to the table or floor if whoever was holding onto it were to let go. One exception: when lying on your stomach, turn your own head from one side to the other any time you feel your neck becoming stiff.

From the moment that you first feel the friend who is giving you the massage make physical contact with your body, try to turn your complete attention to his or her touch. This doesn't mean in any way to analyze it, or to try to figure out what particular technique he or she may be using. On the contrary, simply tune in to the quality of his or her touch the way you might listen to the sound of someone's voice without paying any attention to the meaning of the words.

At the same time continue to keep in touch with your breath throughout the massage. If you want, you can even imagine that your exhalation is flowing to whatever part of your body your friend is working on.

The less said during a massage, the better; during so direct an encounter with your own body, words can only be a distraction. Do feel free to speak up, however, if something that you friend is doing is physically hurting you; or if you feel cold; or if for any other reason you feel uncomfortable. Also, if any time during the massage you should feel a sigh within you, just let it out with the exhalation of your breath.

Finally, when the massage is over you needn't get up immediately. Lie still with your eyes closed; let yourself absorb whatever you are feeling a few minutes longer.

APPLYING OIL

Applying the oil to your friend's body is a simple matter, but there are a few tricks to it worth knowing.

First of all, never pour oil directly from the bottle onto your friend's skin: for many people this is an extremely disagreeable sensation. Put the oil first on your own hands and from there onto your friend's body.

For the same reason be sure that the hand (your own) into which you are pouring the oil is a little to one side of your friend's body, and not directly above it. Then if you should spill a few drops of oil, as does sometimes happen, they won't fall on your friend.

Don't try to pour more than about three quarters of a teaspoon of oil into your hands at one time. Apply this first, and then pour more if you need it.

If the oil is at all cool, warm it in your hands by rubbing them briskly together.

Apply oil only to the part or parts of the body on which you are immediately about to work. Otherwise you will find that your friend's skin has absorbed a part of the oil before you get a chance to use it.

Apply the oil with both palms. Use any kind of simple stroking movement that you want, but make certain that it is both gentle and at the same time very definite and steady. This is especially important the first time you apply oil at the beginning of a massage. It will immediately help your friend to relax if the first impression of your touch is one of confidence and sureness.

Systematically cover the entire area that you are about to massage. Don't miss any corners.

Don't drown your friend's body in oil. Your friend should have no extra puddles of oil visible on his or her skin. About two teaspoons is enough for the average-sized back, for example.

If you do find that you have put on too much oil, you can always remove some of the excess with the backs of your hands or your forearms. Or you can spread some of the oil to another part of your friend's body.

A hairy chest — or leg or back — does require extra oil. Otherwise you will pull the hairs as you move your hands over the surface of the skin.

Be careful where you put down your oil bottle after pouring some oil. If you are working on the floor, try to find a place where it will be easy to find next time you need it and where you won't kick it over. If working on a table, try if possible not to put it anywhere on the table itself: sooner or later this results either in your knocking it over, or in your cramping your movements in order to keep from knocking it over. Much the easier way is to establish one or two convenient nearby places for the bottle before ever beginning the massage.

Here's a problem. One general rule of massage is that once you have first made contact with your friend's body you should try always to have at least one hand touching him or her until the massage is finished. But, as you can see, this presents a difficulty when you are ready to apply more oil: how do you hold your hand to one side of your friend's body when pouring the oil and yet keep physically in contact? The answer is to rest your elbow or a part of your forearm lightly against your friend's body while holding your hands to the side. This feels clumsy the first time you try it. but becomes easy and natural with practice.

One last hint. It took me several years of stumbling around massage tables to wake up to the fact that using two oil bottles instead of one, and placing one somewhere near one end of the table and one somewhere near the other end, can save a lot of steps and acrobatic stretching.

HOW TO USE YOUR HANDS

Knowing how to be at one with your hands is the core of massage, the one real technique. The more massage you do, the more this knowledge will open itself to you. Hands are subtle, however, and getting acquainted with them takes time. I am still learning about mine. It is hardly an unpleasant task, but I know now it will never come to an end.

What I am going to suggest is just a beginning. I strongly recommend that before giving your first massage you read through these comments and try out the experiment mentioned at their end. But be patient, and don't expect to master everything overnight.

Here are some hints.

Apply pressure when you do massage. Once you actually have learned some strokes, the amount of pressure you will use will vary according to the particular stroke and the part of the body on which it is being used. But some pressure is almost always necessary. It has been my experience that many people first learning massage are nervous, consciously or unconsciously, about the possibility of hurting someone with their hands, and as a result they tend to apply almost no pressure. Don't worry; your friends aren't that fragile. Pressure feels good, as you will see when you yourself are being massaged. Learn to experiment with different pressures. Remember, whenever you are afraid you may be pressing too hard you can always check this out with your friend.

Relax your hands. Keep them as loose and flexible as possible while you are moving them. This is difficult — probably more difficult than it sounds to you — for two reasons. One is that to relax a limb while you are in the act of using it is a lot harder than to relax it while it is lying still. The other is that almost all of us, without being aware of it, carry a great deal of chronic tension in our hands. There are ways of getting rid of this kind of tension; doing massage is itself one excellent way, and in a later part of this book I will mention others. These ways do take time; months often, and sometimes even years. You can start in at once, however, merely by paying attention to your hands and by trying to relax them, even if only a degree or so, whenever they feel to you stiff or tight.

Mold your hands to fit the contours over which they are passing. Although certain techniques require, as you will see, that only a specific part of the hands be used, most massage strokes depend for their effectiveness upon your ability to keep your entire palm and fingers always in contact with the person you are massaging. For example, where possible don't let either the heel of the hand or the ends of the fingers slip into the air as you move from one part of the body to another. When you glide your hand over the hip, shape it exactly to fit the hip. When you move it from the chest to the arm, curve it so that it wraps evenly and smoothly around the shoulder as it passes. Think of the way the water of a stream shapes itself to fit the rocks and hollows in its path.

Maintain an evenness of speed and pressure. Try to eliminate trembling, jerkiness, and unnecessary stops and starts. Make any change of either speed or pressure a gradual one, never increasing or decreasing either too suddenly. Let the movement of your hands be as flowing and smooth as possible.

Don't, however, be afraid to vary both speed and pressure. Rhythm is an essential ingredient of massage. You can use different speeds and different pressures without sacrificing the steadiness of your movements. Variety in massage is a lot like variety in music: changes in tempo help avoid rhythmic monotony.

Explore and define the underlying structure of the body of the person you are massaging. (This is a matter of sensitivity, and is something completely apart from the study of formal anatomy; for some remarks about the latter you may refer to a later chapter of the book.) Make your hand constantly question, make it "listen" to the tissue and bone beneath. Tune in to the texture of the deeper strata of the muscles. Is it thick or thin? Tight or loose? Formless or distinct? Where you encounter bone try to outline its shape. Think of your hands as telling your friend, "This is your hip," "These are the tiny bones of your wrist," "This is the way your knee is shaped." To articulate your friend's body for him or her in this fashion is one of the most important aspects of a massage. The more precisely you achieve this, the more your friend's pleasure in his or her massage will take on a deep, almost magical quality.

Use your weight rather than your muscles to apply pressure. It is a fiction that you have to be physically powerful to do massage. Whenever you want extra pressure, get it by leaning the weight of your upper body into your hands rather than by straining with the muscles in your arms and wrists. Straining with your muscles will only give you stiff hands, a less flowing quality of movement, and a tired back.

Once you have made contact with your friend's body, try never to break it until the massage that you are giving or the exercise you are doing is completely finished. Many people, when being massaged, experience any interruption of physical contact as psychologically a little disconcerting. Even when you have to put on more oil keep at least a forearm or an elbow touching some part of your friend's body. Remember that your friend, lying still with his eyes closed, will have entered a universe of touch whose one reality is the contact of your hand.

Do massage with your entire body, not just with your hands. By this I don't mean that you should climb onto the table and roll all over your friend, but that your hands will be most alive when their movement is an extension of a more general movement coming from the rest of the body. This movement of the body need not be great; at times it may be so slight that an observer would scarcely be aware of it. Visible or not, however, you yourself should be able to feel it present as a sort of core from which the more exact movements of your hands are emerging. In some respects the experience of giving a massage is like that of dancing. As with dance, the more total the involvement of the body, the better the massage.

Pay attention to how you are standing, sitting or kneeling.
When working at a table I like to stand whenever possible with my feet apart, my knees bent and turned out, and my back straight. When you first try it this stance will feel awkward to you, but its advantages will soon become apparent. Having your feet apart (a couple of feet, when necessary even farther) permits you to easily swing your entire body up and down the length of the table merely by shifting your weight from one foot to the other. Also, lowering yourself by bending at the

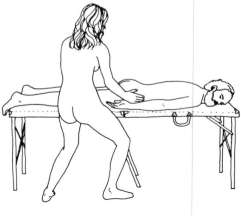

knees rather than bending your back forward eliminates a tremendous amount of potential strain and fatigue in your lower back. And working with a straight rather than a bent back frees your arms and hands for movements that are more controlled and relaxed.

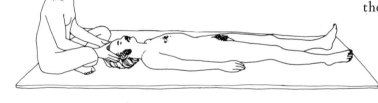

When you are working on the floor the way in which you sit or kneel is largely dictated by the part of the body you are working on, the particular stroke you wish to use, and the like. However, because working on the floor requires more bending of your own back and is therefore more tiring, you must remain all the more aware of the position of your own body.

Try when you sit or kneel to keep your own back straight whenever possible. Also make sure, as I have already stressed, that you have some kind of padding under yourself as well as under your friend. In other words, take care of yourself all you can. The attention you give to your own comfort will be translated to your friend as increased grace and precision in the movement of your hands.

Remember always that you are massaging a person and not an intricate muscle-and-bone machine. Muscle and bone we are, but person too; and we are person throughout every physical cubic inch of us. Your friend is his or her body, as you are yours. Stay aware of this at all times, and keep your hands aware of it; it will have a direct and critical influence on the quality of your touch. About all this there is of course much more to say, and I will discuss these things further in a later chapter.

In order to make these suggestions more concrete here is an experiment that you might try. Have a friend lie down on his (or her) stomach and apply oil to the entire back side of his body. Then put the palms of both your hands against his skin, and start moving them. Don't worry at all about whether they are doing some or another orthodox massage stroke; just move them up and down your friend's body however you wish. Explore how present, how "right there" it is possible for you to feel in your hands. Have your eyes sometimes open, sometimes closed. From time to time experiment with some of what has been suggested above. Try out different pressures, different speeds, and any other changes in quality that suggest themselves to you. Be as spontaneous as you can; let your hands do most of the thinking. At the same time stay alert to exactly what is happening.

Try this for five minutes, ten minutes, or whatever feels good to you, but do it for only as long as you enjoy doing it.

Come back to this exercise as often as you like; it can always teach you something new. These are fundamentals of which our "mastery" is always only partial.

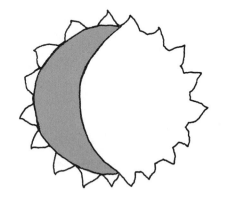

INTRODUCTION TO THE STROKES

Time now to get down to the nitty-gritty of technique. In the section that follows you will find descriptions and illustrations of approximately eighty different massage strokes. Before you start in, however, here are a few necessary bits and pieces of information about how this part of the book has been arranged, about the use of the strokes themselves, and, in case you have never done any massage before, about the best way to go about learning.

The order in which these strokes are presented is not important. If you were to use all of them in sequence, you would end up having given a friend a complete body massage of about an hour and a half in length — a massage that would have started with his or her head, then have worked progressively down the front of the body to the feet, and then (your friend having turned over) up the other side of the body ending on the back. Or, if you were to use only those strokes which I have marked with a star ★, you would give a shorter massage covering the same territory and taking about half the amount of time. The more you experiment, however, the more you will find other, equally good ways to select and combine these various strokes. They are the fundamentals from which your personal massage style will naturally develop.

The particular strokes marked with a star ★ are in no way "better" than the ones not so marked. They merely represent one example of how a short massage can be put together out of the material offered below.

The instructions below have in a sense been written for someone who is right-handed. That is, it is the right rather than the left hand which is favored whenever there is a choice. If you are left-handed, all you have to do is to substitute your left for your right hand in any instances that seem appropriate.

I also generally speak as if you are doing massage on a table: "move to the foot end of the table," etc. In almost all cases, however, what you do if you are working on the floor is exactly the same. Whenever a stroke must be done differently on the floor I have included alternative instructions.

At certain points you will notice that you friend's arm, leg, or head must be lifted or moved. Make sure that you yourself do all the lifting or moving, and that your friend in no way helps out. If he does try to help, or, as sometimes happens, if he slightly stiffens the limb in resistance, just call his attention to it and ask him to relax the limb in question as much as possible.

Learn to make your transitions between strokes seem like a part of the strokes themselves. Even to divide a massage into separate "strokes," as I have done below, is in a certain sense arbitrary. Massage at its best makes use of specific techniques, but only by weaving them into a continuous flowing movement that remains always inventive and spontaneous. Let your hands find a natural way to glide from one stroke into another; your friend should never be able to tell exactly where the one has ended and the other begun. Ideally, in fact, his or her experience of your entire massage should be like that of a single unbroken stroke winding its way all over his or her body.

Remember also, as has already been mentioned, to break physical contact as seldom as possible during a massage. Once you have begun, try always to have at least one hand touching your friend until the massage is completed.

Massage is basically non-verbal and is best done in silence. While you are first making yourself acquainted with techniques, you will of course need to talk with whomever you are massaging in order to find out how he or she is feeling as you work. Other than this, try to focus all your attention on your sense of touch.

If you are learning massage for the first time it is important to go about it in the right way. Here are a few suggestions. My experience is that they can make a big difference in how quickly and easily you learn.

First, a warning! *Don't try to learn too much at one time.* A half dozen strokes or less are plenty for one session. In the beginning you may find massage quite tiring to do.

Very soon, as you learn correctly how to move and position your own body, it will become much less so. But do start with small doses and work up from there!

When you are ready to start in, read over the entire description of a stroke before attempting to do it. An extra reading beforehand of all the strokes you plan to learn at one time will help even more.

Once you do get together with a friend to try out some of the strokes, make sure that your friend gives you as much feedback as possible. Find out what feels good, what bad, what so-so; what feels too light or too heavy; what too fast or too slow; and anything else you want to know. Ask often, and encourage your friend to speak up whenever he or she feels like it. This information will prove invaluable to you.

Experiment especially with different amounts of pressure. Try a stroke lightly, then with more pressure, and then with more pressure still. And ask for feedback at each step.

Don't worry if a stroke at first seems clumsy or awkward to do. Usually if you check out with your friend he or she will have a much different feeling about it.

Finally, whenever possible have the strokes which you are trying to learn done to yourself. You will never really be able to tell how a stroke "works" until you have felt it on your own body. I might add that the nicest way of all to learn massage is with a friend who also wants to learn. That way, you can try out several strokes at a time and he or she can do them on you in turn. This will immediately provide both of you with an "inside" understanding of what you are doing.

Have a good time!

HEAD AND NECK

When I give a complete massage the head is one of my favorite places to begin.

As I have said, the sequence of the different parts of the body that will be followed in these instructions is largely arbitrary. And in a later section of the book I will tell you more specifically about other possible sequences, and why, depending on circumstances, you might want to follow one or another of them.

For now, however, let me say that it is difficult to go wrong in starting out with the head.

The main reason for this is, it seems to me, that having one's head worked on feels like both one of the safest and one of the most startling parts of a good massage. Safest because, in our nervousness about being touched (and we all have at least a residue of this, especially at the very beginning of a massage), it is in the extremities of the body — the head, the hands and the feet — that we least feel the force of our culture's strong taboos against physical contact. And startling because, although the head is the part of the body with which, sadly, we tend most to identify ourselves, it is also one of the parts from which — just as sadly — we feel physically most disconnected. To discover, through massage, that the head belongs to the physical body is a surprise, like awakening from sleep. As a result, by doing his or her head right at the beginning you will provide the friend you are massaging with a good initiation into the deeper and more subtle side of the experience to come.

So let's start.

Stand or kneel so that you are facing the top of your friend's head. Apply a little oil to your fingers, but do not spread the oil on the face prior to beginning. The actual surface of the face is so small that it requires little oil; with the few drops on your fingers you are ready to begin.

The most natural order in which to massage the different parts of the head is first to do the face, starting at the top of the forehead and working systematically down to the chin; then to the ears; the neck; and finally the scalp.

Remember, a star ★ marking a stroke means not that it is better than any of others, but that it is a part of the short massage as described on page

1 Before anything else I like to hold my palms lightly against my friend's forehead for a few moments. Cover the forehead with the heels of your hands, letting the fingers extend down the temples. Apply no pressure. Pause as long as seems right and comfortable to you; a few seconds, half a minute, whatever. Center yourself. Let your friend grow accustomed to your touch.

2 Now begin massaging your friend's forehead with the balls of your thumbs. First mentally divide the forehead into horizontal strips about a half an inch wide. Then, starting with your thumbs at the center of the forehead just below the hairline, glide both thumbs at once in either direction outwards along the topmost strip. Press moderately; use about the pressure it takes to stick a stamp on an envelope. Continue all the way to the temples, a surprisingly sensitive place, and end there by moving your thumbs in a single circle about half an inch wide.

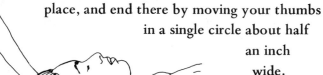

Immediately pick up your thumbs, return them to the center of the forehead, and begin the next strip down, again moving your thumbs from the center outwards. Then, working progressively downwards, do each of the others in turn, ending with a strip running just above your friend's eyebrows. Remember to conclude each strip with another small circle on the temples — a flourish not strictly necessary, but your friend will feel it's very 'right.'

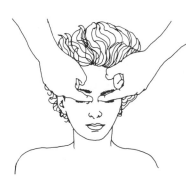

★ **3** The next stroke is for the rim of the eye sockets. With the tips of both forefingers press first against the boney rims of the two eye sockets right where they connect with the nose. Press quite hard for about one full second. Then lift your forefingers, move them about a third of an inch along the upper half of each rim, and press again. Pressing in this fashion is good for the sinuses, and in this particular spot it also feels better to most people than a rubbing movement.

Continue in this fashion, moving about a third of an inch each time you press, until you have reached the outermost point of each eye socket (i.e., the point farthest from the nose). Then return to the point nearest the nose and begin again, this time working the length of the lower half of the rim.

4 Now the eyes themselves. Did you remember to make sure before starting that your friend was not wearing contact lenses? If not, ask about them now.

Lightly run the balls of your thumbs straight across your friend's closed eyelids. Start right beside the nose and move outwards. Go very slowly and use a minimum of pressure, just enough that you can feel the eyeball move ever so slightly as your thumb passes over it.

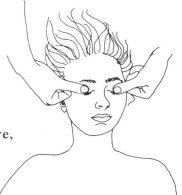

Do this three times, moving your thumbs in the same direction and lifting to return them to the starting point each time.

★ 5 Now place the tips of the forefinger and middle finger on each hand just to either side of the nose, and just below the point on the rim of the eye socket where you started the last stroke. Pressing firmly, draw the tips of these fingers in a path around the

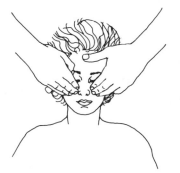

lower edges of the cheekbones, across the cheeks in the direction of the ears, and then back up to the temples for a final circle.

The lower edges of the cheekbones, in case you aren't sure of your geography at this point, lie roughly on a line with the bottom of the nose. If you press firmly and pay attention to the feel of the stroke, however, your fingers will have no difficulty in finding the right place to go.

Do this stroke at least twice. The second time you might want to linger a while on the edges of the cheekbones immediately below and to the sides of the nose, working the muscles beneath by making tiny circles with your fingertips. Let each fingertip move in a circle a quarter of an inch wide or smaller, pressing hard without lifting. Dig in. Don't hurry. This minute area is a focal point for tension in the face, and a little extra work here goes a long way.

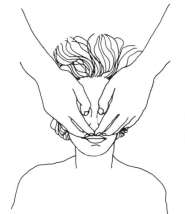

★ 6 Finish the lower half of the face with a series of horizontal strokes like those you did on the forehead.

First use the forefinger and the middle fingers of both hands. Place the tips of these fingers at the center of the face between the nose and the mouth. Stroke outwards onto the cheeks and then up to the temples, ending with the usual circle.

Next do a series of three strokes in the same way between the mouth and the tip of the chin. Start each time at the center and end on the temples.

Then lightly grasp the tip of the chin between the tips of the thumb and forefinger of each hand. Follow the edges of the jaw until you have almost reached the ears, and then glide the forefingers (and the middle fingers too, if you wish) into a last small circle on the temples.

If your friend has a beard, simply go firmly right over it using the same strokes.

This completes the face. Now slide your fingers gently to the ears.

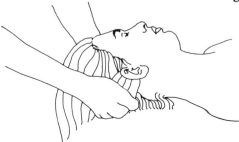

7 Ears seem to me one of the most intriguing parts of the body. I love having mine massaged. Here are a lot of ways to work on them. Use all or any part of this according to your own judgement.

For your first trial run I suggest that you do just one ear at a time. Soon, however, you will find yourself able to do both at once without difficulty.

First run the tips of your fingers several times up and down the back of the ear where it connects with the rest of the head. Move gently and smoothly.

Follow this by gently running the length of your forefinger several times back and forth in the "V" formed by the topmost part of the ear and the skull directly adjacent. Then lightly pinch the outer edge of the ear and the ear lobe between the thumb and forefinger. Start at the lobe right next to the skull and work around, moving your thumb and forefinger about a third of an inch between pinches.

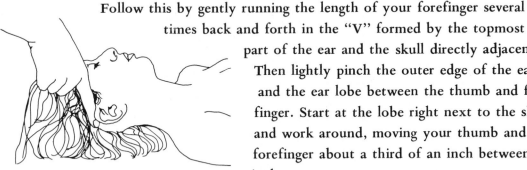

Next, with the tip of the forefinger lightly trace the natural hollows of the inside of the ear. Work from the circumference toward the center. Stop just short of actually closing off the ear channel.

If so far you have been doing just one ear, now do the same steps on the other.

Finally, for the *coup de grace,* tell your friend to listen to the sound inside his head. And then, moving with extreme slowness and gentleness, close both his ear channels with the tips of your forefingers. (Be sure to close both sides at once; nothing will happen if one ear is closed alone.) Keep them closed for about fifteen to thirty seconds. Although some people don't care for this, many enjoy a brief but pleasant journey.

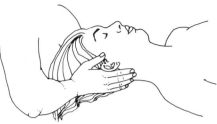

(FROM THE SIDE)

8 This next stroke will feel both odd and awkward as you do it. It is perfectly safe, however, and to your friend will feel extremely good.

Lightly cover your friend's face with both palms, heels of the hands on the forehead and fingertips near the chin. Let your hands rest in place a moment; then slide them gently down, going over and past the ears, until the little fingers of both hands are against the table.

Next begin pressing with both hands as if you were trying to push them together. Make sure your hands are below and in no way pressing on the ears. Crouch slightly and hold your elbows straight out to the side in order to get as much leverage as possible. Start with a gentle pressure and gradually increase it until (unless you are a person of unusual strength) you reach a point at which you are pressing as hard as you can. Then decrease the pressure just as gradually.

After you have released the pressure, hold your hands in place a few seconds more before going on to the next stroke.

Time now to move to the neck.

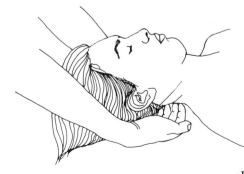

9 Bring both hands palms up under your friend's neck. Then, curving your fingers a little, rapidly drum with the fingertips against the neck. Keep the backs of your hands on the table. Press fairly hard, as if playing a piano. Work up and down the neck, and as far onto the back itself (it won't be very far) in the immediate area of the spine as you can comfortably reach.

10 Next put your hands under the back of your friend's head and gently lift it a little. Then turn it slowly to the left until it rests easily in your left hand. If you sense that your friend is resisting you, or that he is trying to "help," ask him to relax his head as if he were letting it drop to the table. If after this he still has trouble letting go his head, you may be able to help by gently raising and lowering the head a few more times.

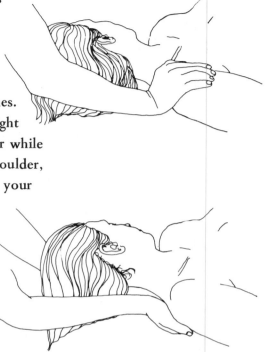

Now slowly rotate the heel of your right hand against the top of your friend's shoulder while bringing your fingers down the side of the shoulder, under the shoulder, and onto the back. Keep your fingers moving across the top of the back towards the spine; and then, just before reaching the spine, onto the back of the neck.

Continue up the back of the neck until your fingertips near your friend's hairline. Then turn your hand about ninety degrees so that your fingers are pointing more upwards (i.e., so that they are perpendicular to the neck itself) and, pressing more lightly, come back down the side of the neck.

Then, moving from the base of the neck, cross the topmost part of the chest straight to the shoulder. From there you can go right into the same stroke again without stopping. Repeat three or four times.

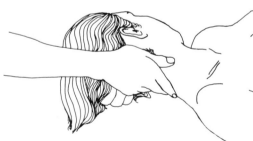

The next two strokes are also done with the head tilted to the side. I prefer to do all three on one side before turning the head and repeating them on the other.

11 With the head still tilted to the left, move the fingers of the right hand in slow circles about an inch wide against the back of the neck. Press firmly. Work up the back of the neck to the hairline. Then, pressing more gently, do circles down the side of the neck, working all the way from just below the ear to the collar bone.   Repeat.

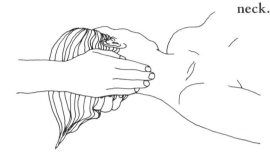

12 Holding your friend's head still turned to the left, find the boney horizontal ridge where the neck meets the back of the skull with the fingertips of your right hand.

Now move your fingertips in tiny circles just below this ridge. Press firmly. You will feel a sort of furrow stretching horizontally across the neck; follow this furrow with your fingertips.

Check in with your friend if you have trouble locating the right place. This is a nice stroke, and he will know at once when you have found the spot.

13 End your work on the neck by lifting your friend's head as far forward as it will go. Use both hands. Move very slowly.

You will feel resistance either soon before or soon after his chin has touched his chest. Stop for a moment when you have reached this point. Then gently nudge his head about an inch farther forward. Bring the head back to the same point, and then push forward once or twice again. If a gentle push isn't enough, then don't push at all.

Again move slowly as you bring the head back down.

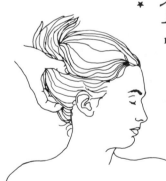

* **14** All that's left now is the scalp.

Again lift the head and turn it to the left. Making your right hand into the shape of a claw, work the scalp on the right side of the head with your fingertips. Press hard, moving your hand in tiny circles. Try to press hard enough that you are moving the skin itself over the bone rather than simply sliding your fingertips back and forth across the surface of the skin. Work systematically (for example, in several wide rows up and down the head) so that you cover the entire right side of the scalp.

Repeat on the other side.

CHEST AND STOMACH

Spread oil on the chest, the stomach, the sides of the torso and the shoulders.

★ 1 Begin the chest and stomach with what I will call the main stroke. Because it covers large areas of body surface easily and quickly, this is one of the most effective strokes in massage. With slight variations it can be done on the chest and stomach, the arm, the front of the leg, the back of the leg, and the back.

Stand above your friend's head. (If working on the floor, kneel above the head with your knees to either side of the head.) Place your hands with palms down in the middle of the chest. Have the heels of your hands resting just below the collarbone, your fingers pointing toward the feet, and your thumbs lightly touching each other.   Now glide both hands slowly forward, pressing firmly on the chest and then more lightly on the stomach. Keep your hands together until you reach the lower half of the stomach; then separate them, moving both hands straight to the sides.

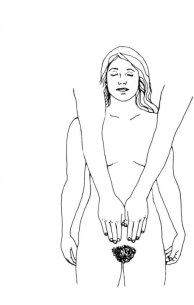

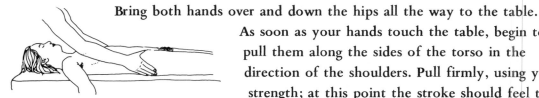

Bring both hands over and down the hips all the way to the table. As soon as your hands touch the table, begin to pull them along the sides of the torso in the direction of the shoulders. Pull firmly, using your strength; at this point the stroke should feel to you as if you were actually about to tug your friend several inches down the table.

Just before reaching the armpits pull your hands — heels of the hands still moving first — up onto the topmost part of the chest. Then, pivoting each hand on its heel, swing the fingertips from the sides to the center of the chest. By gliding the hands forward, and straightening them and bringing the thumbs together as you move, you can go from here straight into another round of the same stroke without breaking the flow of your movement.

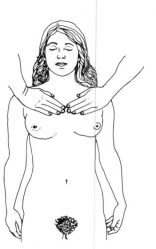

Two reminders that will help make this stroke feel just right. First, be steady. Move at an even and confident pace. Second, remember to mold your hands so that they exactly fit the contours they are passing over. Let your hands tune in to your friend's shape as if you were molding his or her body out of clay.

Here is an interesting variation. After pulling your hands back onto the upper chest, send them over and down the sides of the shoulder instead of pivoting them toward the middle of the chest.

Continue without a break right under the shoulders and onto the topmost part of the back, slipping your fingers between the table and the back.

As soon as your fingers have reached a point right beside — but not directly upon — the spine itself, slide your hands gently over the trapizius muscles (the muscles curving from the neck to the shoulders) and back onto the upper chest.

Another variation, more interesting still. Go down
the sides of the shoulders and onto the back as before.
Again stop just short of the spine. This time, however, pull
your hands lightly onto the back of the neck and then between
the back of the head and the surface of the table. Keep your
hands moving towards yourself until your fingers are completely
clear of the head. Don't lift the head up; keep
the backs of your hands against the table in

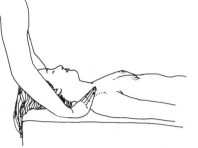

order to disturb the head as little as possible as
you slip your hands from beneath. Once you have
broken contact return your palms immediately to
your friend's chest.

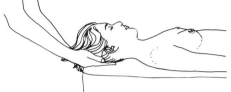

Do the main stroke from three to six times on the
chest and stomach, with or without variations. Occasionally I also repeat it between other strokes
on the chest and stomach; sometimes I even return to it after having gone on to massage other
parts of the body. Returning every once in a while to a major stroke like this one gives a massage
a certain pleasing unity. For both your friend on the table and yourself it can have much the same
effect as the repetition of a basic theme in a piece of music.

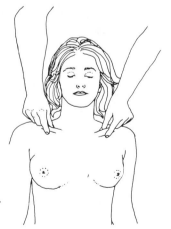

2 Run the tips of the thumb and forefinger of both hands
several times along the collar bone. Have the thumb on one
side of the bone and the forefinger on the other. Move your hands
first toward each other and then away from each other. Press lightly.

★ 3 Work the upper chest with the fingertips of both hands. Press firmly, moving the fingertips in tiny circles. Start next to the collarbone and work systematically so that you cover the entire upper half of the chest. Omit the breasts for a woman, however, as this stroke does not feel good here.

★ 4 Professional masseurs usually do not massage a woman's breasts. Most women I know consider this both prudish and condescending. If your friend is a woman, here is a good stroke for the breasts and the muscles supporting them.
Cup both hands over the breasts. Very gently rotate the breasts as far as you can easily move them in three full circles moving to the right, and then in another three circles moving to the left.

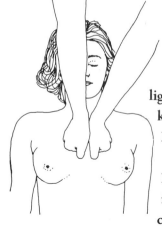

5 Now make both hands into fists. Starting at the middle of the chest just below the collar bone, slide the knuckles of both fists outward across the chest and then down the sides of the torso to the table. Press lightly. Follow the ribs. Try, if you can, to let individual knuckles glide between individual ribs.

Do successive horizontal strips in this fashion until you have covered the entire rib cage. Stop short of the stomach. Remember to go lightly; hard pressure will make this stroke feel terrible. If your friend is a woman, when you get to the central portion of the rib cage do just the two inches or so of ribs between the breasts.

★ 6 This stroke is called pulling, and it is done along the sides of the torso.

Move around to one side of the table and reach across to the opposite side of your friend's torso. With your fingers pointing straight down pull each hand alternately straight up from the table. With each stroke begin pulling with one hand just before the other is about to finish so that there is no break between strokes.

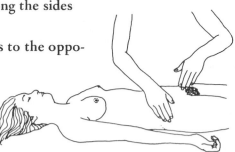

Start on the side of the pelvis just above the thigh and work your way slowly up to the armpit and then back again, moving a little less than the width of one of your hands with each stroke.

Once up the side and then down again is enough. Cross to the other side of the table and repeat on your friend's other side.

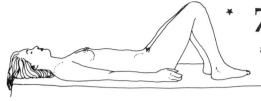

7 Move now to the stomach. Walk around to your friend's right side if you aren't there already, making sure to keep one hand in contact as you move.

The various organs in the stomach area will be less constricted — and hence what you do on the stomach will feel better — if your friend has his knees in the air while you are working directly on the stomach. There are two ways of going about this. The first is simply to place your friend's legs in the right position and then let him balance there himself; by sliding his foot back and forth a little you will quickly find a natural point at which the legs almost balance themselves. The second way is to raise the legs and put a pillow folded in half underneath them for support. I usually do it the first way simply because I don't like to hassle with a pillow in the middle of a massage. The second way, however, does have the slight advantage that your friend doesn't have to siphon off even a fraction of his energy in order to keep his legs in place.

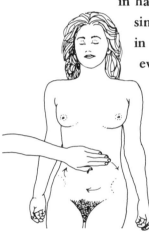

Now stand at your friend's right side and begin slow full circles on the stomach using the palm of your left hand. Move clockwise — most important on the stomach, as the colon is coiled clockwise. With each circle pass first just below the ribs, then a little onto the left side of the torso at the waist, then just above the pelvic bone, and then a little onto the right side of the torso at the waist.

After one complete circle you can add the right hand. Keep the left hand moving steadily in the same fashion; after it has passed from the lower to the upper half of the stomach, however, add the right hand for about a half of a circle running from hip to hip alongside the pelvic bone. As soon as the right hand has reached the right hip, remove it and position it in the air near the left hip so that it can repeat the same crescent movement after the left hand has made another round. Work out the timing so that whenever the right hand is actually massaging, it is at a point on the circle directly opposite to the left hand.

Do a half dozen continuous circles with your left hand, adding a partial circle with the right each time.

8 Awkward as this one may seem at first, in the long run it will be a lot easier for you to do then for me to describe.

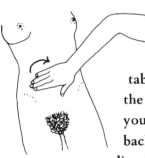

Place the back of your right hand — that's right, the back of the hand — flat against the center of your friend's stomach. Have your wrist bent at a ninety degree angle; your finger-tips should be pointing toward you and your forearm should stick straight into the air with the elbow pointing away from you.

Now start rotating your hand clockwise. After you have completed about a quarter of a circle start gradually turning your hand over onto its palm at the same time; this will also necessarily bring your elbow closer to the level of the table. Keep on rotating and keep on turning, however; so that by the time the circle has been completed, your hand has again been turned onto its back and your elbow raised to a position directly above your hand.

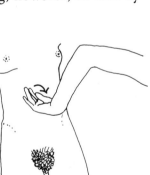

Make half a dozen circles. The feel of this stroke should be flowing and steady and slow. Don't wander about the stomach; keep it right at the center.

If your friend's knees have been raised you may gently return his legs now to the table.

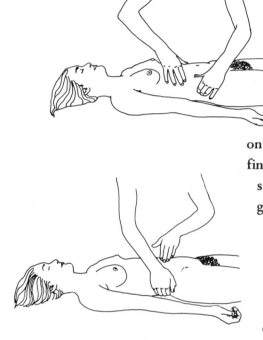

9 Now knead the sides of the torso in the vicinity of the waistline.

Kneading is not difficult. Reach across to the side opposite you. With each stroke of your hands gently squeeze the loose flesh at the waistline between your thumb and fingers; grasp as much as you can comfortably hold onto and then let it slowly slip from between your fingers. Also move your hands a little with each stroke, left hand going to the right and right hand going to the left. If you alternate hands, beginning a new stroke with one hand slightly before finishing a stroke with the other, you will find yourself falling into a slow, lazy, natural rhythm in which the hands are always in motion.

After a few rounds in this fashion you can introduce a change into the stroke. Change your kneading into simple stroking, and instead of moving your hands horizontally (i.e., parallel to the table) along the sides of the torso, begin sliding your fingers under your friend's back right at the waist and drawing your hand vertically up the side of the torso and an inch or two onto the stomach. Follow the waistline and press slightly with the fingertips. Start each stroke from points progressively farther under the back, and start the last two or three from just beside the spine itself.

The shift from the first to the second version of this stroke need not be abrupt. Try doing three or four rounds running horizontally from hip to ribs and back; and then gradually make your strokes more and more vertical until you end with one or two rounds running along the waistline itself.

Then around to the opposite side of the table and do the same on your friend's other side.

10 This last stroke is actually for the back, but it feels nicest when done immediately after the previous stroke.

Reach both hands under your friend's back, one from one side and one from the other, right at the waistline. Palms up, fingers pointing towards each other. Bring the fingertips just to either side of the spine.

Now, keeping the backs of the hands against the table, press the fingertips of both hands as hard as you can just to either side of the spine. Press hard enough to actually raise the middle of your friend's body a tiny bit into the air. Press for about one full second and release. Then again for a second and release. Then again. After the third time or so, slide your hands, still pressing with the fingertips but pressing much more lightly now, out from under the back and, again following the waist- line, onto the stomach. As with the previous stroke, articulate the waistline as you go.

If you are working on the floor, here is — at last — one place where you have an advantage over someone working on a table. After (or even instead of) pressing your fingertips next to the spine, squat so that you are straddling your friend's body, lace your fingers together behind the spine itself, and lift the middle of your friend's body several inches off the floor. Then slide your hands along the waistline, pressing slightly with the fingertips, as you let your friend down again. For your friend, the sensation of being lifted will give this stroke an especially pleasant feeling.

Don't bother with this variation, however, if you are working on a table. Because you are forced to reach from the side it's both more tiring for your own back and more difficult to do correctly.

Whichever version of this stroke you are using, a nice way to finish is to keep following the waistline with your fingertips until your hands meet at the center of the stomach. Go more lightly while crossing the stomach itself. Once your hands meet, you can then find some graceful way to glide them to wherever you plan next to work.

THE ARM

Arrange your friend's right arm at his side with the palm turned down against the table. Spread oil on the arm and shoulder.

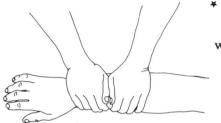

★ **1** Begin with a variation of the main stroke. Place both your hands palms down across your friend's wrist, cupping them so that they cover the sides as well as the top of the wrist. Have your hands side by side, with thumbs touching.

Pressing firmly, glide both hands together up the arm. Separate them only when you reach the top of the arm, sending the left hand over the top of the shoulder and the right down the inside of the arm just short of the armpit.

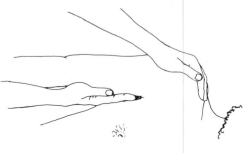

Now pull both hands back down the arm, starting with your left hand on the outside and your right on the inside. Press more lightly. Once you reach the wrist you have two options. One is simply to slide your left hand around onto the top of the wrist so that both hands are in position to begin the same stroke again.

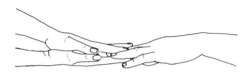

The other, if you feel like something with more of a flourish, is to slide both hands down the length of your friend's hand and right off his or her fingertips. Let your right hand slide along the top of the hand and your left hand the bottom.

Press more lightly on the hand, and be extra delicate and precise as you leave the fingertips. Immediately afterwards move your hands into position for your next stroke so that your friend experiences as little a break in contact as possible.

* 2 This stroke is called draining.

Raise your friend's forearm so that it is standing upright with the elbow still against the table. Now make a ring around your friend's wrist with the thumbs and forefingers of both your hands; tilt your hands away from you so that your palms are facing up as you hold the wrist. Have your thumbs against the inside of the wrist, and have both thumbs touching each other.

Now, squeezing lightly with your thumbs and forefingers, slide both hands slowly down the length of the forearm as if you were "draining" it. When you reach the crook of the elbow slide both hands back up again, still keeping your thumbs and forefingers in contact with the skin but now applying no pressure at all. Repeat several times.

Why, you may ask, do we use pressure going down but not coming up? The answer is that the veins, which lie closer to the surface of the skin than the arteries, are more immediately affected by external pressure. Hence when we "massage towards the heart," as a traditional bit of massage lore puts it, we are giving an extra push to the blood circulating through the veins towards the heart. For many of the other strokes I am describing to you this traditional rule does not greatly matter. When draining the forearm, however, a little experimentation will soon convince you that your friend will be happiest when you apply pressure going down — but not up as well.

* 3 Keep your friend's forearm in the same upright position.

Placing the fingers of both hands against the back of your friend's wrist for leverage, begin massaging the inside of his wrist with the balls of your thumbs. Use your thumbs alternately, and send each stroke downward and out toward one or the other side of the wrist. Gradually work your hands downwards until you have covered all the muscles lying along the inside of the forearm.

4 A quick treat in passing for the elbow.
First, with your friend's forearm still upright, make a loose fist with one hand and lightly massage the crook of his arm — the inside part of the elbow area — with your knuckles. This is a tender area, so be gentle.

Next, lift the upper arm a little off the table with one hand, and, using the tips of the thumb and fingers of your other hand, massage the boney surface of the elbow itself. Work in tiny circles over the entire elbow.

★ 5 Now repeat strokes 2 and 3 on the upper arm. You will find that keeping the upper arm in a steady vertical position can be a bit of a problem, however.   One solution is to place his hand on your own left shoulder and to press your cheek against it, much as if you were holding a violin in place.

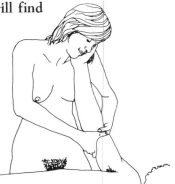

A second is to bend his arm at the elbow and to let the forearm dangle across his body at about the level of the neck. If you use this position take care not to slap the forearm against his chin while you are working on the upper arm.   Taking your pick of these two positions, first drain the upper arm and then work the exposed muscles with your thumbs just as you did for the forearm.

6 Next hold the entire arm straight upright. With your right hand grasp the wrist; with your left push horizontally against the elbow to keep the arm from bending in the middle.   Now, keeping it vertical and unbending, bob the arm lightly up and down in its socket. Press down and then immediately release the pressure a half dozen times or so in quick succession.

7 Your friend's arm is still standing straight upright, right? Now toss it from side to side.

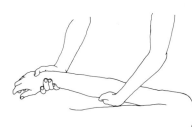

Lower the arm first to the right (i.e., towards your friend's hip), still holding the wrist with your right hand and the elbow with your left.

Then lightly toss it up and to the left, keeping your hands in contact. As soon as it starts to fall to the left (i.e., towards your friend's head), switch your hands, raising the left hand to the wrist and lowering the right to the elbow, so that you now can break the fall with your left hand. Let the arm fall almost to the table and then toss it again, this time to the right.

Switch hands again as it is falling to the right, and you are ready to repeat the entire sequence.

If your friend's arm feels stiff, and does not fall naturally and easily, remind him to let go of it.

Toss the arm three times back and forth.

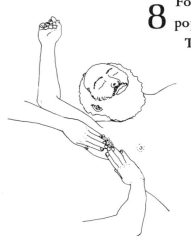

8 For a last goodby to the arm here is an especially nice stroke made popular by Molly Day Schackman.

Toss the right arm one more time (see the previous stroke, in case you have been following a different sequence) to the left, catch it, and then let it rest in place, the upper arm on the table beside the head and the forearm partially resting in the air. Meanwhile place both your palms lightly against your friend's armpit area, with the fingers of either hand pointing towards the other.

Now begin spreading your hands to the sides, leading with the heels of the hands. Start with a light pressure. Send the right hand down the side of the torso and the left along the upper arm.

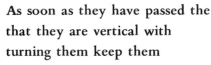

As soon as they have passed the
that they are vertical with
turning them keep them
At the same
with your left hand,
thumb below, and curve
that the full palm presses
as it passes.
Keep both hands in this
them apart. Increase the pressure
reaches your friend's hip and your

armpit itself turn both hands so
respect to the table; while
moving apart at the same pace.
time lightly grasp the arm
fingers on top of the arm and
your right hand a little so
against the side of the torso

position as you continue moving
slightly. Stop when your right hand
left reaches his wrist.

Now, keeping your hands in place, hold more tightly and stretch the arm and the hip away from each other. Hold this stretch for about one full second, and then release, breaking contact just long enough to bring your hands back to your friend's armpit.

Repeat the entire stroke one more time. A moment or so after breaking contact the second time, return both hands to the arm itself and gently put it back into place at your friend's side.

I prefer to massage both the right arm and hand before going on to the left arm and hand. If you have just finished your friend's right arm, you may wish to go on to the following section on the hand before moving over to his or her left arm and hand.

THE HAND

The hand requires very little oil. What you have left on your own hands after massaging the arm will be more than sufficient.

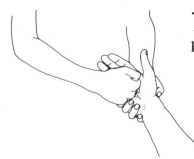

1 First place your friend's hand palm in the palm of your own left hand. Make a fist with your right hand and massage the palm with your knuckles. Move the knuckles in circles a half an inch to an inch wide. Press firmly. Cover the entire palm without moving onto the fingers.

* 2 Next go over the same area using the tips of your thumbs. Hold the back of the hand with your fingers and press hard with the thumbs, moving them also in small circles. This time, however, continue up over the heel of the hand and, pressing more gently, an inch or so onto the inside of the wrist.

Want to try something more elaborate? Do this stroke on the palm (but not the wrist) while holding your friend's hand as follows. Have your friend's hand palm up. Place the little finger of your left hand between his forefinger and middle finger; the fourth and middle finger of your left hand between his forefinger and thumb; and the forefinger of your left hand on the other side of his thumb. At the same time place the little finger of your right hand between his middle and fourth fingers; the fourth finger of your right hand between his fourth and little fingers; and the middle finger and forefinger of your right hand on the other side of his little finger.

Got that?

Now push all your fingers as far onto the back of his hand as you can. Then push your fingers hard *against* the back of his hand. See what this does? If you are pushing correctly you will have bent his fingers back so that the entire surface of his palm is stretched taut as a drum. And now, keeping his fingers bent back, begin working the palm with the tips of your thumbs. Press hard, and go patiently into every tiniest nook and cranny. As you will find out the first time it is done to you, this stroke is more than worth the extra effort.

* 3 Now work the back of the hand with the tips of your thumbs. Be thorough. Go also an inch onto the wrist, paying particular attention to all the tiny bones your thumbs will find there.

4 For this stroke you will have to follow some anatomical guidelines.

Hold your friend's hand palm down in your own left hand, and for a moment study the back of his hand. Notice the small raised cords, just under the surface of the skin, that appear to run from the base of the wrist to the first knuckle of each finger. These are actually the tendons that are used to extend the fingers. (If you have difficulty locating them try looking at the back of your own hand by itself while stretching your fingers as far out and back as they will reach. This will raise the tendons and make them more visible.)

Now, thinking of these tendons as ridges and of the spaces in between as valleys, slowly run the tip of your thumb down each valley in turn. Go all the way from the base of the wrist to the little flap of skin between each successive pair of fingers. Use enough pressure that your friend can feel each valley as perfectly distinct; use a little less, however, as soon as you reach the flap of skin between the fingers. Do each valley one time, using your right thumb for the two valleys nearest the right side of the hand and your left thumb for the two valleys nearest the left.

Here is a flourish you can add, if you feel so moved, each time your thumb reaches the little flap of skin between two fingers. Press the underside of the flap with the tip of your forefinger as your thumb begins to press from above, by this means giving a gentle pinch to the skin as your thumb and forefinger slide off it. It will make a nice stroke feel even nicer.

5 Although a little difficult at first, this stroke is quite simple once you get the knack of it.

Hold your friend's hand palm down with both your hands. Have the heels of your hand pressing against the middle of the back of his hand, and the tips of your fingers press- ing against the middle of the palm underneath. Have the heels of your hands touching each other, and the corresponding fingers of both hands also touch- ing one another.

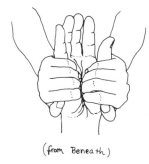

(from Beneath)

Now begin pressing very hard upwards with your fingertips and downwards with the heels of your hands. At the same time begin very slowly sliding the heels of your hands from the middle of the hand to both edges. Stop when the heels of your hands are at the edges of your friend's hand.

Do this stroke three times.

6 Now do the fingers themselves.

Hold your friend's hand palm down in your left hand. With your own thumb and forefinger lightly grasp his thumb where it joins with the rest of his hand. Now slide your thumb and forefinger slowly from base to top of the thumb, twisting your hand from side to side in a corkscrew motion at the same time. Pull a little as you go. End by going right off the tip of the thumb into the air.

Do each finger once in the same way.

7 Here is a nice way to finish your work on the hand.

For a minute hold your friend's hand sandwiched between both of yours. Make contact with as much of its surface as you can. Be still, go inside yourself, and concentrate on your own breathing. Then focus your attention back onto your friend's hand and try to let the energy of your breath seep from your own hands into that of your friend.

This pause need not be long — thirty seconds is fine. Afterwards you will find yourself refreshed, and your friend will have opened himself a little more to what is yet to come.

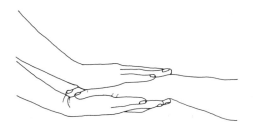

FRONT OF THE LEG

See that your friend's feet are a foot or so apart. Apply oil to the entirety of the front and sides of the right leg.

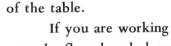

★ **1** For the main stroke on the leg, it is important to stand or kneel in exactly the right place. If you are using a table stand near your friend's right foreleg and turn forty-five degrees toward the opposite end of the table; in other words you should be roughly facing the pelvic region of your friend's body. Have your weight on your right foot and place your left foot a couple of feet toward the head of the table.

If you are working on the floor kneel alongside your friend's foreleg. Be facing in the direction of your friend's head; have your knees approximately parallel to his or her knees.

Now place your right hand across your friend's ankle with fingertips facing your side of the table. Place your left hand just in front of the right with fingertips facing the opposite side of the table. (If you are working on the left leg the right hand goes in front of the left hand.) Both hands should be cupped, with fingers together; the thumb of the left hand should be resting against the little finger of the right.

Now glide both hands from one end of the leg to the other. The movement should be slow and steady. Go lightly over the knee but elsewhere use plenty of pressure; this can be most easily done by leaning slightly over the leg and thus using the natural effect of your own weight rather than an increased muscular effort. If you are standing, transfer your weight from your right to your left foot as you move. If kneeling, you may, if you wish, raise yourself slightly upwards and forwards in order to keep the upper part of your own body directly above your hands as long as possible.

The trickiest part of the stroke comes when you reach the top of your friend's leg. Here the hands divide and go their separate ways.

The left hand continues upwards until the finger tips find the hip bone. It then follows the line of the hip all the way down to the table; as it does so, the fingertips with a slight extra pressure outline the curve of the bone itself.

Then, once the fingertips have actually made contact with the table, the left hand begins to move along the side of the leg back toward the foot.

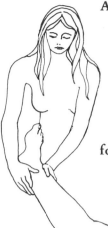

At the same time the right hand moves more slowly down the inside of the thigh. There is a natural crease in the skin between the pelvis and the inside of the thigh; the fingertips should follow this crease, making a detour around a male's genitals where necessary, straight down to the table. At this point the right hand is also ready to head back toward the foot.

Now as you gradually transfer your weight back onto your right foot, pull both hands along the sides of the legs all the way to the ankle. Keep the fingertips on both sides moving against or just above the surface of the table. Use less pressure than going up; however, let your friend feel a definite pull as your hands move down.

When you move your hands into place to repeat the stroke be sure to end up with the left hand higher up on the foreleg than the right. Otherwise the hands will be in each other's way when it is time for them to divide. For the same reason, when you later move to your friend's left leg you must there place your right hand higher up than your left.

I find that there are two secrets to making this stroke feel exactly right. The first is to articulate the hip bone as carefully and as precisely as possible with the left hand. For your friend this will feel as if you are drawing a picture of his body's structure at this point, a sensation which most people find particularly pleasant. The second secret is to pace the movement of the two hands, after they have divided at the top of the leg, so that they end up parallel to one another when they begin their downward journey back toward the calf. This means that the inside hand must move considerably more slowly than the outside one. You can, of course, just move it at the same speed and then let it rest in place until the left catches up. The stroke feels nicest, however, if you can somehow work it out so that both hands stay constantly in motion.

A nice variation: move the hands up the leg as before, but coming down use just your fingertips and make the pressure as light as possible — as if you were stroking the skin with feathers. This feels exquisite, as I urge you to verify the next time you are the lucky one on the table.

Repeat the main stroke three or more times. I like also to include it now and then between some of the other strokes that I use on the front of the leg.

2 For the next stroke, place the palm of your left hand flat against the outer side of your friend's foreleg. Have the hand halfway between the ankle and the knee, with the fingertips pointing towards the knee. Now, looking at the inner side of your friend's foreleg, picture this side as divided into three parallel strips running from ankle to knee. Place your right hand at the ankle end of the topmost strip with finger tips pointing toward the knee.

Then, holding the left hand in place, slowly glide the right hand along this topmost strip until the fingertips are just short of the knee. Then bring it back to the ankle, leading now with the heel of the hand, without any change in the speed or pressure of your stroke. The left hand stays in place the whole time. However, it exerts pressure in opposition to the moving right hand so that the muscles of the foreleg are gently squeezed between.

After covering the first strip once both forwards and backwards, do the next two strips in succession. Then place the right hand flat against the inner side of the foreleg, and with the left hand do three strips in exactly the same fashion on the outer side.

Next move to the thigh (or, if you prefer, to our next stroke for the knee and then to the thigh) and follow the same sequence. However, since the thigh is wider you will here have to do four or more strips on each side. On the inner side let each strip run from a point parallel to the knee to the crease in the skin between thigh and pelvis. The strips on the outer side should also begin at a point parallel to the knee, but should go on to include the hip as well; let the fingertips of the left hand make contact with the edge of the hip bone each time before returning.

★ **3** Now the knee! This is one of my favorites. Your friend may well discover for the first time what a pleasure it can be to have a knee. Although it looks complicated, the stroke is fairly simple. First I am going to break it down for you into halves. Begin by placing the crossed tips of both thumbs against the lower edge of the kneecap.

Next with the tip of the left thumb circle the edge of the kneecap. Move to the right (in other words, counter-clockwise), and make a complete circle. You will find a small furrow between the edge of the kneecap and the bone underneath; press the tip of the thumb into this furrow with a light but steady pressure. Then do the same thing with the right thumb, this time starting to the left, or clockwise.

Now for the actual stroke, merely move both thumbs at once exactly as you moved them separately. First bring them up either side, then let them cross at the top, and then finish by bringing each thumb down the side opposite that from which it started. At the bottom of the kneecap cross them again and you are ready to begin another circle. Do three or more slow circles without lifting your thumbs or stopping.

Afterwards drum lightly all over the top of the kneecap for several seconds with the fingertips of both hands. Finish by gently rubbing the sides of the knee with the fingers of both hands at once. Make half a dozen or so wide circles on either side of the knee.

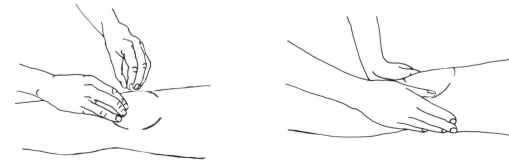

4 For the next two strokes your friend's leg must be raised so that the knee rests in the air. Lift with your left hand from beneath the knee while with your right hand you slide the foot until it is parallel to the knee of the opposite leg; the knee should be high enough that the leg is almost able to balance in place. Next, if working on a table, anchor the leg in place by backing up and sitting so that you gently pin your friend's toes under your own right buttock. If you are working on the floor, kneel and hold his foot between your own knees.

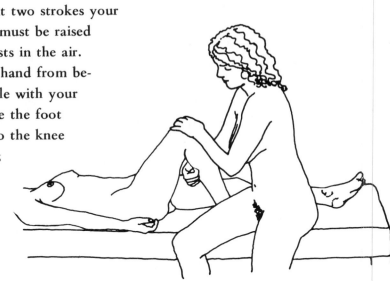

Now, lightly clenching your right fist, reach under the leg from the right and with the inside of your forearm massage the calf muscles on the underside of your friend's foreleg. Starting with the inside of your wrist at the base of the calf, work in long narrow circles going first from left to right. As you come up the left (from where you are facing) side of the calf, keep sliding your forearm to the left so that by the time you have made it to the top of the calf you have almost reached the crook of your elbow.

Coming down again on the right side, slide your forearm back to the right until the inside of your wrist is once more against the base of your friend's calf.

Circle two more times in the same direction, then another three times in the opposite direction. Give this stroke your best attention: it is also one of everybody's favorites.

5 This one is called "rolling" the thigh. Leave your friend's leg in the same raised position that you used for the previous stroke.

Place your palms on either side of the thigh just below the knee, your fingers extended outwards. Now vigorously move both hands back and forth, moving the left hand forward (i.e., in the direction of its own fingertips) while the right hand moves back (i.e., in the direction of its own heel), and vice versa; and at the same time slowly work both hands down the length of the thigh.

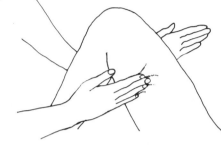

Continue down the thigh almost to the pelvis, and then return upward with the same motion. Repeat the entire stroke one more time.

As with the arm and hand, I like to massage both the right leg and the right foot before going on to the left leg and foot. If you wish to do the same, follow your work on the right leg by going on to the next section for the foot.

THE FOOT

If any single part of the body deserves your best attention it is the foot.

Psychologically it is the point at which we experience our connection with the ground that supports us. It is where we feel, if and when we are lucky enough to do so, that we are "rooted."

From a bone and muscle point of view, moreover, it is an unusually delicate and complicated piece of equipment. If you could strip off your skin you would find twenty-six separate bones making up the skeletal machinery of one foot alone.

But what counts most for those of us doing massage is the role the foot plays within the nervous system of the body. In the sole of the foot are concentrated literally tens of thousands of nerve endings, and the opposite ends of these nerves are located all over the rest of the body.

Thus the foot is a "map" of the entire body. No muscle, no gland, no organ whether internal or external, is without a set of nerves whose opposite ends are anchored in the foot. And what does this mean? Simply that when we massage the foot we stimulate and affect all the rest of the body as well: So critical, in fact, are these groups of nervous correspondences between the foot and everything else in the body, that an important means of medical diagnosis and healing through foot massage, commonly called "zone therapy" by practitioners, has been built entirely upon it. I will have more to say about zone therapy in a later section. Enough for now that you be aware that while massaging the foot you are giving an extra "shadow massage" to the rest of the body as well. So do good work — a little here goes a long way.

The strokes for the foot are much like those for the hand. Also like the hand, the foot requires little oil. Whatever you have on your hands after massaging the leg will most likely be enough.

1 First make a fist with your right hand. Steady the foot with your left hand, and with the knuckles of your right hand massage the sole. Move your knuckles in small circles; press hard. Be sure to cover the entire sole, including the bottom of the heel.

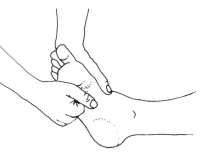

★ **2** Next go over the sole with the thumbs of both hands. Hold the foot in place with your fingers and work both thumbs at once in small circles. Again cover the entire sole. Go slow. Be thorough. Remember those thousands of nerves connecting the foot with the rest of the body.

If you are working on the floor you will find this one of the more awkward strokes of the massage. One thing to do that can help: sit cross-legged facing in the direction of your friend's head and rest the foot or the back of the ankle on your own knee or leg. Another way: prop the foot up on a thick cushion or pillow.

★ **3** Next work the top of the foot, using your thumbs in the same way. Again be vigorous and be thorough; don't let any tiny patches escape unmassaged. When you reach the lower half of the foot — in other words when you near the ankle and the heel — you will find it easier to use the tips of your fingers. Circle the ankle bone itself — the round bony protuberance about the width of a half dollar on either side of the ankle — several times with your fingertips, doing both sides at once.

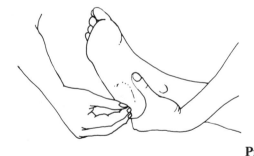

4 When you finally reach the lower end of the heel, gently lift the foot from beneath the ankle with the left hand and work the bottommost edge of the heel with the tips of the fingers and thumb of the right hand. Press hard.

5 Next look at the top of your friend's foot and find, just as you did for the hand, the long thin tendons running from the base of the ankle to each toe. Run the tip of your thumb, pressing firmly, down each of the valleys that lie in between these tendons. Start at the base of the ankle and end at the tiny flap of skin between the toes. As for the hand, you may, if you wish, gently squeeze this flap of skin by pressing the tip of your forefinger against its underside as your thumb passes over its top. Do each valley one time.

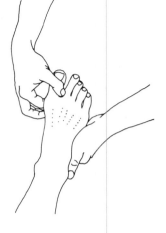

6 Next squeeze the foot just as you did the hand. Grasp the foot with both hands, heels of the hands against the top of the foot and fingertips pressing into the middle of the sole. Have the heels of your hands touching each other, and the corresponding fingers of both hands also touching one another.

Now begin pressing very hard downwards onto the top of the foot with the heels of your hands and upwards into the sole with your fingertips. At the same time very slowly let the heels of your hands slip from the middle of the foot out to either edge. Stop right at either edge.

Do three times.

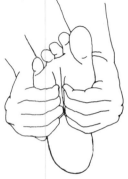

(from Beneath)

★ 7 Now the toes themselves. With your left hand hold the foot steady; with the thumb and forefinger of your right hand grasp the base of the big toe. Then gently pull, twisting from side to side in a in a corkscrew motion, until your thumb and forefinger slide off the tip of the toe. Do each toe in turn.

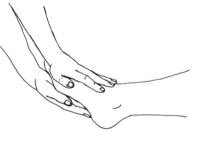

★ 8 Finish the foot just as you did the hand. Clasp the foot between your hands, one palm along the sole and the other along the length of the top, and for a moment allow yourself to be still. Center yourself and become aware of your breathing. Imagine that you're sending your breath into your hands, allowing the energy that circulates in your own body to mingle with that of your friend's.

BACK OF THE LEG

If you are following the sequence I have used in describing the strokes, it is time to have your friend turn over onto his stomach. Remember to keep one hand in contact as he moves. Have him lie with his head turned to whichever side he wishes, and remind him to turn his head to the other side whenever his neck feels tired.

Spread oil on your friend's right leg, buttock and hip.

★ **1** Begin with the main stroke. The version for the back of the leg is almost exactly like the one for the front of the leg. Place your friend's feet a foot or so apart. Stand beside your friend's right foot. Place your left hand across the back of the ankle with fingertips pointing toward yourself, and your right hand just above with fingertips pointing toward the opposite side of the table. Pressing firmly, move both hands together up the leg; go more lightly, however, over the back of the knee. Remember to transfer your weight from your left to your right foot as you move.

Separate your hands at the top of the thigh just as you did on the front of the leg. Send the right hand over the top of the buttock until the fingertips locate the hip bone. Glide the hand down the hip to the table, firmly articulating the curve of the bone, and then bring it along side of the leg back toward the foot.

At the same time move the left hand more slowly down the inside of the thigh. Try to work out the timing (as with the front of the leg, this will take a little practice) so that the left hand arrives at the lowest point it can comfortably reach on the inside of the thigh just as the right hand, coming off the hip, passes into a position directly parallel to it. Then pull both hands along the sides of the leg all the way back to the ankle. As your hands near the ankle, try to return them to the starting position of the stroke without a break in the flow of your movement.

Repeat this stroke three or more times, and return to it as often as you like between the strokes to follow.

2 Remember the "Indian burn" when you were a kid? Here is a version of the Indian burn that feels as good as the old one felt bad. In massage we call it "wringing."

Cup both hands and place them, with fingertips pointing away from you, side by side across the base of your friend's calf. Have the underside of the fingers and as much of the palms as possible in contact with the leg.

Now let's first look at the stroke in slow motion. Move your left hand away from you and down, maintaining full contact with the leg, until the fingertips reach the table. At the same time move your right hand towards you and down, until the heel of the hand also reaches the table.

Next move both hands all the way in the reverse direction, ending with the heel of the left hand and the fingertips of the right against the table. Then move both hands back to the opposite position. And so forth.

Now speed up this movement and you have "wringing." Keep both hands crossing rapidly back and forth, and at the same time work them together slowly up the length of the leg. The crossing movement, though light in pressure, should be as fast and vigorous as you can make it without sacrificing definiteness. Keep the hands always crossing in directions opposite to each other, and keep the thumbs always brushing against each other.

Continue the stroke all the way to the top of the leg and back down again. One time up and back is enough.

3 Next we "drain" the leg just as we earlier "drained" the arm.

Place your palms against either side of the foreleg right at the ankle. Have as much of the palms as possible in contact with the leg, with fingers either touching or pointing toward the table on a slant of about forty-five degrees. Across the base of the calf place both thumbs, pointing in opposite directions and touching each other.

Now slowly glide both hands up the foreleg, squeezing gently with palms and thumbs alike. Stop just before you reach the knee and then, moving at the same slow pace but this time with no pressure, glide the hands back down the length of the foreleg. The thumbs remain touching each other throughout the movement.

Go up and back three times, applying pressure each time during the upward movement only. Then move to the thigh and, starting just above the knee, do the same stroke three more times. As you near the pelvis the width of your friend's thigh will probably force your thumbs apart. Simply bring them together again on the way back down.

★ 4 Next use the balls of your thumbs to massage the thick muscles of the calf. Press firmly, moving your thumbs away from you in short, alternating strokes. Cover all the back of the foreleg.

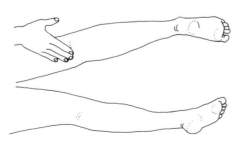

5 With the fingers of one hand lightly massage the slightly hollow area in back of the knee. Work your fingers in small, gentle circles.

6 ★ Next comes "pulling" on the inside of the thigh. Beginning on the inside of the thigh just past the knee, pull your hands upwards in slow alternating vertical strokes. Keep the palms in contact with the skin, and the fingers pointing toward the table. Begin each new stroke just as you are finishing the previous one. Keep the pressure gentle, and the rhythm slow and steady.

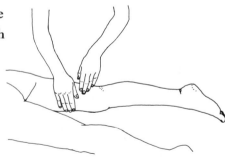

Start each stroke a little higher up the leg (i.e., farther from the knee), until you reach a point just short of the pelvis. Then slowly work back down toward the knee in the same fashion.

If your friend had his or her way you would probably keep doing this stroke all afternoon, but twice up and back is sufficient.

7 Next try "raking." This is a good stroke almost anywhere, but I particularly like to use it on the back of the leg, the buttocks, and the back itself.

Hold each hand with the fingers spread apart and slightly curved. Stiffen the fingers a little. Each hand should now look like a claw.

Now begin working down the length of the leg with short alternating strokes. Begin at the top of the leg or, if you want, on the buttock itself. Keep both hands in the claw position, and use only the fingertips for actual contact. Work rapidly and with a very firm pressure, making each stroke about six inches long.

Go systematically down the entire leg, trying to cover as much as you can of the sides as well as the back of the leg. Work downwards only; for some reason this stroke doesn't feel good when done in the opposite direction.

As soon as you have reached the ankle, start again at back to the top of the leg and repeat one more time.

8 Finish by lifting the foreleg and bending it back toward the buttock. Find the point at which the foreleg resists being pushed back, and then, *gently* nudging it an inch or two further, bounce it several times in this position. Push the heel of the foot against the buttock if you can do so without straining. Then lower the leg slowly back to the table.

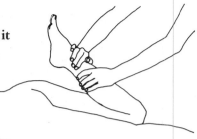

THE BUTTOCKS

The buttocks are the easiest part of the body to massage. Not the least of reasons for this fact is that here almost anything you do feels good.

★ **1** Begin by kneading the flesh of either buttock exactly as if you were preparing bread for the oven. Lift the flesh and squeeze it between the thumb and the other fingers. Knead rhythmically, alternating hands. First cover one buttock thoroughly and then go on to the other. Moving from one to the other side of the table isn't necessary; you can knead either buttock from where you stand.

2 For the next stroke consider the buttocks to go all the way from the waistline to the tops of the thighs.
Stand at your friend's left side. Hold the middle three fingers of your right hand (or your left if you are lefthanded) tightly together so that the tips form a triangle with the middle finger on top, and place these three fingertips at a point just below your friend's waistline and just to the right of his spine. Pressing firmly, begin working your fingertips in circles a half an inch wide or smaller, and at the same time slowly move your hand toward the opposite side of the table.

Continue to make circles in this fashion, following an imaginary strip running straight across and then down the side of the buttock (or what in this case you might call the lower back) until your fingers reach the table. Then with almost no pressure slide the fingertips in a straight line back up the same strip.

Continue working across and down the side of the buttock in strips of this kind. Let each strip begin about an inch farther down the buttock; start each one just beside the spine, or, once you have run out of spine, just above the groove between the buttocks; each time slide back up the same strip once your fingers have reached the table. Work all the way down the right buttock and then cross to the other side of the table and do the same for the left.

3 The next stroke is not difficult, but finding the exact spot to do it can be a little tricky.

With the fingertips of one hand lightly probe the flesh roughly an inch to the side of the center of the buttock. What you are looking for is a slight hollow or indentation between two large folds of muscle, the Gluteus medius and the Gluteus maximus. Usually it is more readily felt with the fingers than seen with the eyes. If you can't find it, don't worry. Either your friend is a freak, or you may simply need a little more practice. In either case just go ahead with the stroke at any point that looks to you like it ought to have been the proper spot. It will still feel reasonably pleasant.

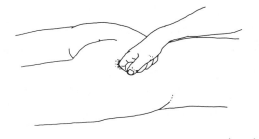

Now double up one forefinger, press its second knuckle into this hollow, and slowly turn your hand as far as you can in either direction. Turn three times each way and then stop. That much feels quite pleasant, but more may make your friend imagine that he is being bolted to the table.

This stroke of course should be repeated on the other buttock. I prefer, however, to go on and do the following stroke on the same buttock, and then to cross over and repeat both on the other.

4 If you never found that hollow, here's your second chance. Back to the same spot, this time with the heel of your hand. Point the fingers up into the air and press the heel straight into the hollow. Now vibrate your hand as fast as you can; try to make your whole arm tremble and shake as if you were getting an electric shock.

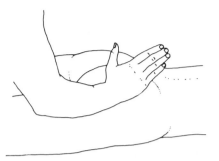

After ten seconds or so of vibrating your hand in place, start moving the heel of your hand over the rest of the buttock. Keep pressing, keep vibrating. In order to be systematic about covering the entire territory, I would suggest that you divide the buttock again into one inch wide strips. This time, however, think of the strips as running up and down instead of across the buttock. Start with the strip running next to the groove between the buttocks and end with the one bordering upon the table. Move your hand up (i.e., toward the head) one strip and down (i.e., toward the feet) the next.

★ 5 Now for the simplest stroke of our massage. Spread the fingers of your right hand as wide apart as you can, and then place your hand firmly against the lower slopes of both buttocks at once. Now shake your hand lightly but very quickly from side to side, shaking the buttocks beneath at the same time. Looks silly? Just ask your friend how it feels.

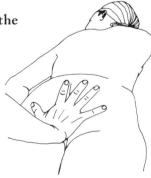

THE BACK

According to the yogis of India and Tibet, our psychological and spiritual condition is more dependent on the state of the spine than on any other part of the body. I am inclined to believe this is correct for a number of reasons, not the least of which is the deep sense of release most of us feel when the back is properly and thoroughly massaged. Because of its importance as well as its size, I would suggest that you spend more time working on the back than on any other single part of the body.

Spread oil on the back, the shoulders, and the sides of the torso. Also the buttocks if you have not worked on them just previously.

★ **1** Begin with the main stroke on the back.
One nice thing about the main stroke on the back is that it can be done in either direction.

If you are working on a table the easiest way to do it is from a standing position at the end of the table above your friend's head.

If you are working on the floor, however, you have two choices open to you. One is to sit or kneel just above your friend's head and to do the stroke exactly as described for working on a table. The other is to sit straddling your friend's thighs — a very comfortable position from which to work and to run the stroke in the reverse direction. If you want to do the latter, read through and try to understand the first way of doing it before attempting it in the opposite direction.

Here's the first way. Stand or sit above your friend's head. Place your palms on either side of the topmost part of the back with fingers pointing toward the spine. Have the tips of your fingers right beside, but not on, the spine itself; like many others for the back, this stroke feels much less pleasant if allowed to wander directly onto the spine.

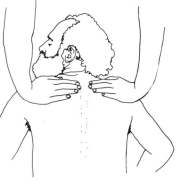

Now glide your hands down the entire length of the back. Maintain a firm pressure, leaning forward to use as much as possible of your own weight. Press extra hard with your fingertips. You will be able to feel a small furrow just to either side of the spine; let your fingertips press right into these furrows as they pass.

Separate the hands when you near the lower end of the spine, leading the hands over and down the sides of the hips until they touch the table. Then slowly pull both hands along the sides of the torso in the direction of the shoulders. Pull hard, almost hard enough to move your friend on the table. Just before reaching the armpits, glide your hands once more onto the topmost part of the back. Then pivot them, turning the fingers toward the spine, so that they are in place to repeat the entire stroke.

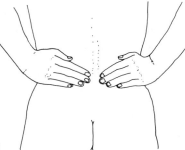

A good variation of this stroke is to take both hands all the way over the tops of the buttocks before pulling them back along the sides. In general it is a nice idea, when doing strokes for the back, to include the buttocks whenever you can.

If you are working on the floor and prefer to sit straddling your friend's thighs, just start with your hands on the lower back with fingertips pointing towards the spine. Take your hands straight up the back; separate them at the top of the back, bringing them over the shoulder blades and down to the table; and then pull them back down along the sides. And if you want to make it all feel even better, let your fingertips outline the tops of the shoulder blades when your hands separate at the top of the back. Use a little extra pressure with your fingertips and they will pick up a natural curving groove that they can follow all the way from the spine to the shoulders themselves.

Do the main stroke on the back from four to six times, repeating it whenever you wish between other strokes as well.

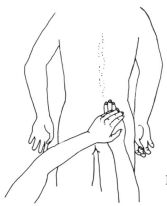

2 Now stand on either side of the table beside your friend's lower back. Or, if you are working on the floor and have decided to sit straddling your friend's thighs, you may continue from the same position.

Place your right hand on your friend's lower back just to the right of the spine. Have the fingertips of the hand right at the waistline and pointing toward the head. Then place your left hand palm down on top of your right.

Now make a circle with both hands around the hip bone. Follow the waistline straight to the table, go several inches down the hip (i.e., toward the feet), cross up onto the top of the buttock, and from there go back to the waistline beside the spine. Lean your weight into your hands and use plenty of pressure.

Repeat this circle at least four times. Then do the same on the other side of the lower back, again starting at the waistline just beside the spine and this time circling your hands to the left.

This is an important stroke, by the way, since the lower back is a high tension area for almost everyone.

★ 3 Now work with your thumbs on the lower back. Using the balls of your thumbs, make short rapid alternating strokes moving away from you. Let both thumbs go over the same spot at least several times before moving on. Work close to the spine just below the waistline, in an area about the size of a large grapefruit.

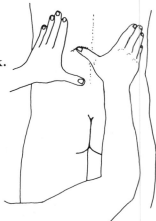

★ 4 The "rocking horse." One stroke that actually does go up and down the spine itself. Stand at your friend's left side. Place your right hand on your friend's spine, heel at the lower end of the spine and fingers pointing towards the head. Place your left hand on top of and across your right, fingers pointing toward the far side of the table.

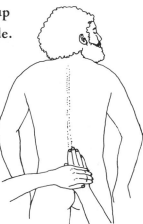

Now slowly glide both hands straight up the spine. Keep the pressure moderate and steady.

As soon as you reach the top of the back, start down again at the same speed. As you come down, however, lift your right hand slightly so that it is no longer touching the spine and at the same time dig the tips of your right forefinger and middle finger into the two furrows that lie immediately to either side of the spine. Glide both fingertips straight down these two furrows, pressing as hard as you can. If you bend both fingers as much as possible at the joints closest to the tips, you will maximize the downward pressure at the tips themselves.

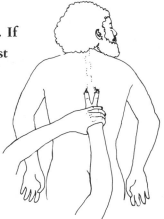

Go all the way down to the lower end of the spine and an inch or two more onto the buttocks. Widen the distance between your fingers when you come onto the buttocks, as if you were tracing an upside-down "V."

The Anne Kent Rush variation of the rocking horse is one of the great strokes in massage. Go up the spine as usual. Take your left hand away from your right, however, as soon as you reach the top of the back. Then with the right hand begin coming down as before, digging the tips of the forefinger and the middle finger into the two furrows to either side of the spine. Only bring it just four inches or so down the spine and then take it away. Meanwhile do the same thing with the left hand, starting about an inch farther down from where the right hand started; begin pressing with the left forefinger and middle finger slightly before the right forefinger and middle finger have broken contact. Then begin stroking again with the right hand, this time starting an inch down from where the left hand started; and so on. Work this way down the full spine, overlapping your strokes and starting each a little lower on the spine. Your friend will experience this as waves flowing down his or her entire back.

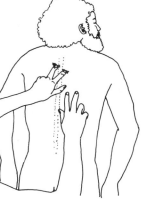

Do the rocking horse two or three times.

5 Now do pulling along the sides of the torso, just as you did when you were working on the chest and stomach. Reach across the table and work the side opposite you. (If you are working on the floor and are straddling your friend's thighs, this stroke can be done from where you are sitting. Just lean a little to the right as you massage the left side of your friend's torso, and vice versa.)

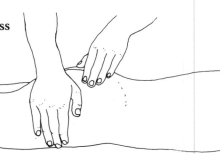

Start just above the thigh, and work up to the armpit and then back again. Pull each hand straight up from the table, keeping the fingers pointing downward. Find a slow hand-over-hand rhythm, letting each new stroke begin just as the one before is about to finish.

Work once up and then down again on both sides of the torso.

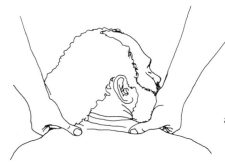

6 Now we move to the upper back, frequently another high tension area. Begin by kneading the muscles curving from your friend's neck onto his or her shoulders. Work the muscles gently between the thumb and fingers. Do both sides at once.

7 Next the shoulder blades.

This is a great stroke, by the way, but is extremely awkward to do without a table. If you are working on the floor you may well want to skip this one and go straight onto the next stroke for the upper back.

The first problem is to raise one of the blades so that the surrounding muscles are made more accessible. Standing at your friend's right side (if you are working on a table you may actually find it easier to kneel while doing this stroke), take his right hand and place it palm up in the middle of his back. Then lift his shoulder an inch or two from the table and slide your 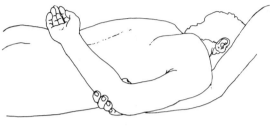 own right forearm, underside up, under the shoulder; let the shoulder come to rest right at the crook of your elbow; and then with your right hand clasp your friend's forearm (if you can't reach it, don't worry about it) near his elbow. Now the blade is raised and you are ready to go to work.

The key area to massage is the furrow running around three sides (top, side nearest the spine, and bottom) of the now raised blade. First run the fingertips of your left hand several times slowly back and forth along all three sides. Be firm; strong pressure feels good here.

Next make tiny circles with your fingertips, again going several times along all three sides. Dig in, going very slowly and making your circles a quarter of an inch wide or even smaller.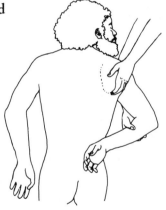

Then, to finish, shape your left hand as if it were a claw, pressing firmly on the blade itself, try actually to move the skin over the blade in circles. Go several times to the right, then several times to the left. Then slide your hand lightly down the length of your friend's arm, put his hand and arm back on the table, and gently extract your own forearm from under his shoulder.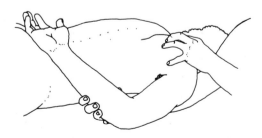

Do the same on the other side.

8 Now use your thumbs on the upper back just as you did on the lower back. Stand above your friend's head. Move your thumbs away from you in short and rapid alternating strokes. Stay off both the spine and the shoulder blades themselves. Concentrate first on the muscles just above the blades, then on those lying between the blades and the spine.

9 The "corkscrew." Easy once you get the hang of it. Stand on either side of the table. Place your right hand on his right shoulder, left hand on his left. Have the fingers of both hands pointing towards the table.

Now slowly pull both hands, heels first, toward the spine. Press as you pull. When the hands are about to meet, swing each hand 180º around so that the fingers end up pointing in the opposite direction. Keep both hands moving at the same pace the whole time, left hand moving to the right and right hand to the left; your forearms will cross as your hands pass the spine.

Continue moving the hands across the back until the fingertips of both hands have simultaneously reached the table. At the same time lead both hands a little lower down the back (i.e., in the direction of the feet); so that the right hand touches the table just below the left armpit, and the left hand just below the right armpit.

Start gliding your hands back again toward the spine the moment your fingers have made contact with the table. As before, begin by moving them heels first; then pivot them 180° in the middle of the back, uncrossing your forearms as you do so; and end by sending the right hand fingers first to the table on the right side, and the left hand the same way on the left. Also, as before, bring them about three inches farther down the back.

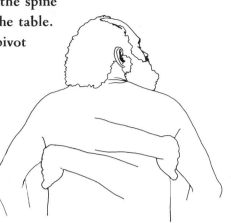

Continue in this fashion, crossing and uncrossing your arms and moving a little lower down the back each time your hands go from one side to the other. Stop when your hands have reached a point roughly abreast of the lower end of the spine. Then head up the back again in the same way, ending with your hands once more on the shoulders.

Once down and back up again is enough.

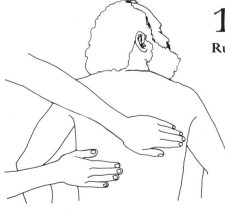

10 Here is the equivalent of "wringing" (stroke 2 for the back of the leg) for the back. Run your palms in speedy horizontal strips across the back. Pull your right hand toward yourself as you push your left hand away from yourself, and vice versa. Keep the hands moving constantly, rapidly, and without ever leaving the surface of the skin; generate as much friction as you can. Keep off the sides of the torso — this would slow you down too much.

Starting at the top of the back, work gradually down the length of the spine and back up again.

Once down and back is sufficient; especially since this stroke, if you are doing it right, is tiring for you if continued very long.

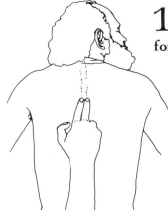

11 This one is more subtle than it looks.
Trace your friend's spine from neck to tail bone with the forefinger and middle finger of one hand. Start where the neck meets the base of the skull. Use the tips of the two fingers. Keep the pressure moderate and move very slowly, letting your fingers take in the particular texture of each vertebra in turn.

That's all.

*12 Finish with this one.
Place the undersides of both your forearms straight across your friend's back halfway between the top of the back and the lower end of the buttocks. Have your forearms as close

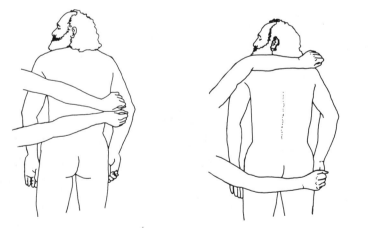

together as you can, and tilt your hands back so that the skin on the underside of your forearms is stretched a little.

Now slowly spread your forearms apart, pressing hard. Keep them moving at the same pace until one forearm has reached the top of the back and the other has crossed the buttocks. Then lift them off the surface of the skin, instantly return them to the middle of the back, and repeat the stroke.

After two passes over the spine itself, lean a little over the table, slant your forearms slightly downward, and do the same stroke along the far side of the back. Then readjust your position and do the same along the near side of the back. Then, starting again at the center but this time working at an angle, do the stroke diagonally so that one forearm ends at the shoulder nearer you and the other passes over the buttock on the opposite side. Then conclude with a second diagonal stroke, this time going to the far shoulder and the near buttock.

A superb stroke, this is an especially nice one for ending your work on the back.

FULL-LENGTH STROKES

The best way to end a massage is with a few good strokes running up and down the full length of the body. Besides being fun for you to do, such strokes will leave your friend with a deeper awareness of his body as a connected whole.

1 Do "raking" as described earlier for stroke 7 on the back of the leg. This time work down the length of the back, over the buttocks, and continue all the way down one leg. Then again down the back, the buttocks and all the way down the other leg.

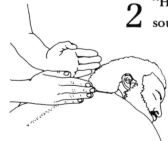

2 "Hacking," a stroke which feels better than its name sounds, was the one being done the last time you saw someone getting a massage in a Hollywood movie.

Drum the outer edges of the hands lightly, but as rapidly as possible, against the spine. Start at the top of the spine and work downwards; continue moving at the same pace all the way down one leg. Then work back up the length of the body, retracing the same path. Then repeat, this time going down and back up the other leg.

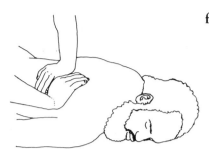

3 Now glide both hands up one leg as if you were going to do the main stroke for the back of the leg (see stroke 1 for the back of the leg). But this time don't divide the hands at the top of the leg.

Instead, continue without a break right over the buttock and up one side of the back.

Separate the hands and pivot them only when you have reached the top of the shoulder blade on the same side of the body. Then bring them heels first down the side and leg, all the way back to the ankle. Don't go onto the spine.

Repeat once or twice more. Then go around the table and do the same on the other side.

4 This one is called the "bear walk." I have heard it claimed that to this day, in some of the most rural villages of Eastern Europe, for a few coins you can lie on the ground and have a trained bear administer the authentic version of this stroke.

Reach across the table and press one palm against the top three inches or so of the farther side of your friend's back. Have the heel of your hand just to the far side of his spine. Press very hard, leaning as much of your weight into your hand as you can. Next press your other hand right beside the first — in other words, immediately below it on your friend's back — again taking care to place the heel of your hand just to the far side of the spine. Then cross your first hand over and press it immediately below the second, and so on. Begin pressing with one hand just as you release the pressure of the other. Walk the bear all the way down the side of the back, over the buttock, and down the leg; and then (having crossed over to the other side of the table) up the other leg, the other buttock, and the other side of the back. Press as hard as you can each time. One exception; press much more lightly on the backs of the knees.

5 If you spread the thumb and forefinger of one hand as far apart as possible, the skin between the two becomes taut. This creates a versatile tool for massage. The next stroke is done entirely with these few inches of stretched skin. Stand at your friend's left side. Run the spread thumb and forefinger of your right hand all the way up the left leg, over the buttock, and up the left side of the back. Press hard, move rapidly, and use only the thumb, the forefinger, and the 'V' of skin stretched between. Go lightly over the back of the knee.

As you near the top of the back begin bringing the left hand — thumb and forefinger spread in the same fashion — back down the same route. Then again up the full

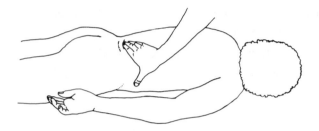

length of the body with the right hand, then again back down with the left, and so on.

If your own feet are spread several feet apart (or, when working on the floor, if you spread your knees as far apart as you can), you can weave your entire body back and forth along with the movement of your hands. A lively and forceful stroke, this one can be particularly enjoyable to do.

Go up and down a half a dozen times or so. Then, naturally, the same on the other side.

6 Now try the main stroke going up both legs at once. Stand at one side of the table near your friend's feet and stretch yourself a little over the table. Place your right hand across the back of your friend's right ankle, fingers pointing inward; and your left hand across the back of your friend's left ankle, fingers also pointing inward.

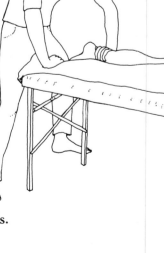

Go right up both legs, over the buttocks, and up the back. Walk a little with the stroke if necessary. Coming down, pull both hands down the sides of the torso, over the hips, and down the outer sides of the two legs. Keep the movement even and steady, and try, if possible, to exert an equal amount of pressure with both hands.

Go at least three times up and down.

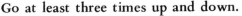

I might add that Stroke 6 is one stroke that actually is a lot easier if you are working on the floor. All you have to do is to kneel between your friend's legs and do the entire stroke from there. If I am feeling dexterous and don't think I will unnerve whomever I am massaging, once in a while I even climb up onto my massage table in order to do this stroke at the right pace and with the right evenness of pressure.

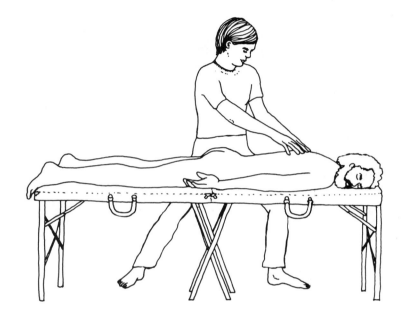

★ 7 Using both hands at once, do a series of feather-light strokes straight down from the head and neck to the feet. Use only the tips of your fingers, and go as lightly as you can without actually leaving the surface of the skin.

For a change of texture you can also use your nails a few times. By curving your fingers a lot you can bring your nails into play no matter how short they are. Before you finish, however, for at least a moment go back to feather-light stroking with your fingertips.

Be soft, slow, and subtle. By now your friend is likely to be so relaxed that your least touch will seem rich and full.

★ **8** The chief thing about the Last Stroke is to do it carefully. It always leaves a lingering impression.

One possibility: take a final feather-light stroke down the length of the body and precisely off both feet at once.

Another: glide your hands down your friend's arms, and then hold your palms lightly against his or her hands for a little while before breaking contact.

Another: have your friend turn over, massage his or her face once more, and then hold your palms lightly against his forehead for a little while. This is especially nice if you began the massage this way.

After you have taken your hands away do not disturb your friend for at least several minutes. Move quietly. Cover him with a sheet if you suspect that he might be cold. (Remember that a room feels about five degrees colder if your skin is oiled.) If you like to be still and inside yourself for a few moments after completing a massage, now is a good opportunity.

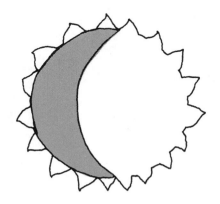

OTHER SEQUENCES

When you are giving a complete massage, in what order or sequence ought you to work on the different parts of the body? Ask five different masseurs or masseuses (a masseur is a man who does massage, a masseuse a woman) and you will get five different opinions. My own feeling, after much experimentation with different orders and combinations, is that there is no "ought." In fact the one recommendation I would make is that you vary the sequence which you follow as much as you can. Both for yourself, and for those of your subjects who have already had some experience with massage, this will go a long way toward keeping what you are doing from feeling habitual and stale.

What are the possibilities?

The first question is where to start. I very much like beginning with the head, for reasons which I have mentioned in the instructions on how to massage the head. However, also among my favorite places to begin are the abdomen, since it is physically and psychologically the center of the body; the feet, since they are the part of the body with which many of us are most out of touch; and the back.

Concerning the back there is a little more to say. One practice I do follow is always to begin with the back whenever the person I am about to massage seems nervous or uptight about the massage itself. Like the head, the hands, and the feet, the back is a part of the body where almost everyone feels more safe in being touched. At the same time it provides a particularly large area that is ideally suited to a lot of good massage work. Start on the back, and you can go a long way toward relaxing someone who is nervous. After this, once it comes time to move elsewhere, he or she is likely to experience the other parts of his or her body as feeling much less vulnerable.

I also go straight to the back whenever the same kind of problem occurs during the course of a massage. If the person I am massaging appears suddenly to have become nervous about being touched, I immediately leave the place I have been working and move to the back, having him turn over if necessary. After spending some time on the back I then return to the place I first was working. Almost always the situation has changed for the better.

Another practice I usually follow in determining the sequence of a body parts is to move from one part to another which is immediately adjacent whenever possible. In other words, I massage the hand either just before or just after massaging the arm on the same side, etc. Somehow this seems to make more sense — it feels more "right" — to the person being massaged. Nevertheless, this rule is no more strict than any other, and I myself frequently break it. For example, as an interesting change of pace (either for myself or for a subject who has already received a number of massages) I sometimes begin by massaging both feet and both hands before anything else.

A more obvious convenience, both to you and to the person being massaged, is for you to complete one side of the body before turning to the other. The most common exception: sometimes I like to end a massage by covering one or more parts of the body a second time. Suppose, for example, I have been roughly following the order outlined in the instruction section of this book. At the end I might ask my subject again to turn over onto his back and then once more massage his face — an especially nice way to close. Or I might finish with some additional full-length strokes on the front half of his body.

What about the order of the strokes themselves on any one part of the body? On the whole this is arbitrary; almost any order you follow will do. One nice touch, however, is to both begin and end with strokes that cover the entire body part being worked on — for example, on a leg both begin and end with the main stroke. Also, whenever you find it necessary to divide a body part into several smaller areas — for example, when using separate strokes for the foreleg, the knee and the thigh — it will feel best to your subject if you work systematically from area to adjacent area rather than moving around at random.

Finally, the very principle that you must completely finish one part of the body before going on to another is itself arbitrary. It is true that most people, including most professionals, do massage in this way. But it is not the only way; and, as I am increasingly becoming convinced, it is not even necessarily the best way. I do think it is a good idea to work part by part in the orthodox fashion until you have become quite adept at doing massage. Once you feel ready for it, however, try giving an occasional massage in which you go from one to another body part with every other stroke or so. After a stroke on the leg, for example, move to a stroke to two on the stomach and chest, from there to the arm, then the neck, then back to the chest, and so on. If done with the right smoothness and flow, a massage of this kind will not only keep your subject more sensitive and alert but also give him a more satisfying sense of his body as a connected whole. You will probably also find for yourself that it is more fun to do.

To sum up, the only "right" order to follow while giving a massage is the one which feels the most fitting at the moment. Try never to do exactly the same massage twice.

MAKING UP YOUR OWN STROKES

Making up your own strokes is not hard. The more massage you do, the easier it will become. Your hands, you will find, have tremendous imagination. The secret lies in learning ways to trigger this imagination.

The simplest and most direct method to go about discovering new strokes is every now and then during a massage to stop whatever you have been doing, suspend what you were planning and let your hands try out whatever they want. Ask your hands, not your head. Try to give them as much freedom as possible. They will often surprise you.

Other ways of experimenting can also give you new ideas. One good way is to try to transfer a stroke "meant" for one part of the body onto another part. Sometimes this will work — usually with a lot of changes in the nature of the stroke — and sometimes not. But whether it works or not your hands are likely to discover something new in the process.

Another device is to try to find all the ways you can to massage more than one body part with a single continuous stroke. In other words, find or invent a stroke that includes, e.g., both the back of the leg and the lower back. The obvious way to start doing this is simply to combine two or more strokes that you have already learned. Later, as you get into this kind of thing, you will find yourself becoming more and more innovative.

It can be an additional help to experiment with different ways of moving your hands. Most of the strokes listed in the instruction section of this book are versions of what is classical massage jargon is called "effleurage" — stroking with the full open palm. But a number of other ways of working with your hands can also be put to use on almost any part of the body. Try, for example:
* stroking with the balls of the thumbs (as shown in the instruction section for the inside of the wrist)
* moving the fingertips with deep pressure in tiny circles (as shown for the chest)
* kneading (as shown for the buttocks)
* raking (as shown for the back of the leg)
* stroking with the heels of the hands

* stroking with the undersides of closed fists
* drumming with the fingertips
* hacking (as shown as a full-length stroke)
* large sweeps and circles with the undersides of the forearms (as shown for the back)
* pressing lightly with the elbow (use the flat part of the elbow, not the tip)
* light slapping (best done with the hands cupped)

And you will find others.

Another good device is to seek out every way you can to let your hands articulate and define the muscular and skeletal systems of your subject's body. Let your hands say, "Here this is, and this is how it is shaped" — a muscle group, a curve of a bone, or whatever. Many new ideas will come to you if you try exploring in this manner.

A further help along the same lines: learn some anatony. As you have no doubt noticed, no knowledge of formal anatomy is required for using the strokes given in the instruction section of this book. But the more you learn about the underlying physiological structure of the body, the more you will be able to both refine the techniques presented here and develop new ones of your own. A good way to start is to make yourself thoroughly familiar with the charts in the chapter on anatomy in this book. After that you might try exploring a few textbooks on anatomy, or even taking a course or two on the subject.

New strokes are easy to find. The key is continual experimentation. After all, that's how massage came into being in the first place.

BODY TENSION

What is tension? In the sense in which we are using the word here, it is a stiffness or tightening of the muscles and the connective tissue beyond the amount of tonus needed for normal healthy functioning. Its origin is mostly, and possibly entirely, emotional in nature, and the greater part of it is chronic, which is to say that it is with us at all times — even when we are sleeping. As such it is a constant drain (although often a subconscious one) upon our vitality. When it is released, we normally experience a surge of heightened energy.

Whenever you are about to massage a friend try to study the patterns of tension in his or her body before he or she climbs onto the massage table. This takes practice but once you have done a certain amount of massage you will be surprised how easy it can be to "read" another person's body.

One important set of clues is to be found in the person's general physical posture. For example:

Are your friend's shoulders too high? Hunched forward? Held rigidly back? Is either shoulder pulled up higher than the other? Is either pulled in closer to the neck, making that half of the torso appear smaller than the other half?

His head, looked at from the side — thrust forward? Held back? Either is an indication of tension in the neck.

Does his face, or any part of it, appear pinched and tight?

His back, looked at from the side — how wide or narrow is the "S" of its curve? Wideness in the top part of the "S" indicates tension in the shoulders and upper back; wideness in the lower part, tension in the pelvis and lower back.

Another set of clues can be found in the way your friend moves and uses his body. Is he naturally mobile and expressive, or does he tend to "hold himself in?" Do some parts of his body appear vital and active, while others parts are left rigid and unused? Are his gestures easy and flowing, or more sharp and staccato? Does his face easily reflect the flow of his emotions, or does it appear constricted and immobile?

Once your friend is undressed and lying on the table you can learn still more.

For example, do all parts of his body appear to sink down into the table, or with some or all does he appear to hold himself a tiny bit up from it?

If he is lying on his back, do his feet lean a little outwards, or are they pointing rigidly upright? If the latter, look for tension in legs and hips.

Do his hips look tight, turned in?

Do his hands look as if he is about to make a fist with them?

Does his chest look tight and pulled in?

The color of the skin provides another set of clues. Wherever it appears whiter and more faded, look in that area of the body for a greater amount of tension.

Take a look also at the movement of the breath in the body. If the breath is shallow and makes itself visible more in his chest than his abdomen, look for a lot of tension in the entire torso and the neck as well.

After you have looked with your eyes, the next step is to "look" with your hands. This, of course, is most easily done during the massage itself. In the long run you will find that by touching another person you can tell even more about the patterns of muscular tension in his body than you can by looking at him.

What do your hands "look" for? Here there is less than I can tell you. In a particularly tight area — especially in the upper back just above and beside the shoulder blades — your fingers are likely to find tiny lumps, anywhere from the size of a pea up, buried under the flesh; normally these are either deposits of waste matter or knottings of the connective tissue. In general, however, where someone's body is tense the flesh simply feels tight, feels stiff and resistant to your handling of it. Being able to sense this with any precision is a skill you will develop only by doing a lot of massage on a number of different people with different body types. Pay attention to the variations you find from person to person, and your hands will gradually get the knack of it.

Once you have located tension in a person's body, what do you do about it?

The first thing is to massage a much wider area than just that of the tension itself. The reason for this is that the place which either you or your subject have found is actually only the focal point of a larger, more diffused pattern of tension.

The next step is to do some good massage work directly on the focal point or points themselves. Use strokes with plenty of pressure; the best are those using either the tips of your fingers or the balls of your thumbs, as these concentrate the pressure of your hands in a much smaller area. Go slowly and systematically, tuning in all you can to any minute changes that may be taking place in the muscles and tissue on which are are working.

In some regions of the body — especially around the upper back, the shoulders and the neck — you will find that when you are working on a tense area even a moderate degree of pressure may cause your friend a small amount of pain. If so, tell your friend that this is a "good hurt" and that he will immediately feel better when you stop. Don't, however, press extremely hard (i.e., with all or most of your body weight) on a place that hurts; not that is, unless you have had either a lot of experience doing massage or the chance to study deep massage with a teacher. Extremely hard pressure can in fact be a useful tool for working on tension of this sort, but you must know exactly what you are doing when you use it.

The occasion is rare, but you will sometimes encounter a subject with a lot of body tension who will get up off your table and discover that he feels more tense after the massage than he did before! What has happened is this. In all of us tension exists in layers, and we frequently use a surface layer of tension to cut ourselves off from any awareness of the deeper layers beneath. A good massage may reduce much of this surface layer without, however, having been able to have as great an effect upon the other layers below. This means that the deeper layers may now make themselves fully felt for the first time. The person will actually have considerably less total tension but, having been made more aware of what is really going on in his body, he experiences more tension than before!

One more warning. Never neglect the rest of the body for the sake of one or two areas of higher tension. Do economize, cutting down on the amount of time you might have spent on one part of the body in order to spend more on a more tense part; but don't economize too much. The living tissue of the body is an interconnected whole, a single envelope whose various parts are much more dependent upon and responsive to one another than is commonly realized. For reducing tension, and for every other aspect of massage as well, the one rule before all others is: deal with the body as a whole.

NERVOUSNESS, DISCOMFORT AND THE TICKLES

Excessive nervousness, physical discomfort on the table, and ticklishness can all set roadblocks in the path of a good massage. Sometimes these obstacles are insurmountable; usually, however, you can find ways to get around them. Here are a few remedies and countermeasures which you will want to have at hand.

Nervousness during a massage comes in many shapes and varieties. Most people who want a massage in the first place are not particularly afflicted by it. Some people are, however, and among these the most common response is nervousness about being nude.

Fortunately, this is fairly easy to deal with. One simple method is to place a towel over the buttocks when your friend is lying on his (or her) stomach, and over the genitals when he is lying on his back; a second towel can also be placed over a woman's breasts.

A sheet can be used instead of a towel, or in addition to it. This way only that particular body part actually being massaged need be exposed at any one time.

A third solution: have your friend wear either his or her underwear, or a swimming suit. Needless to say, this will drastically cut down on the number of strokes that you can do. However, nudity more than loses its value at that point at which it leaves a subject so tense that he or she cannot enjoy his or her massage.

The other form of nervousness during a massage is an excessive uneasiness about being touched. This fear, while overlapping with the fear of nudity, is different from it and comes from another place in the personality. It is also more difficult to deal with. It manifests itself sometimes as an extreme tightening and pulling in of the body as it is being touched, sometimes as a violent trembling, and sometimes simply as an overt refusal to proceed any further with the massage.

If your friend reacts with this degree of nervousness there is not a great deal that you can do. One possible step, which I have already mentioned in the chapter on sequences, is to leave whatever body part you have been working on and move to the back. Massage done on the back, more than any other single body part, often has an immediate calming effect.

Another approach that can sometimes help is to spend a few minutes working closely with your friend on his breathing. First ask him to feel the weight of his body against the table and leave him alone (i.e., don't touch him) for a minute or two while he does so. Then ask him to follow the movement of his breath within his body, to let his breath, without forcing it, become as long and natural as possible, and to let it flow as deep into his torso as he can manage. Then, after another minute or so has passed, place one of your hands lightly under the nape of his neck and the other on his stomch just below the rib cage. Watch his breath closely, and with the hand on his stomach begin pressing down slightly as he exhales and then releasing the pressure as he inhales. Don't take your hand away at any point; just alternately increase and decrease the pressure without breaking contact.

The idea is to get him to deepen his breath spontaneously. This you can "suggest" to him with your hand. Each time he exhales, continue to press lightly downward a fraction of a second after his exhalation appears to have stopped. And each time he inhales make the pressure of your hand so light that it almost — but not quite — breaks contact. Also, if you see that his breath is beginning to get deeper, try moving your hand a little lower on the stomach. This will lead his breath lower into the pelvis and will help him to relax still further.

At this point you may find that your friend is accepting your touch more calmly and that you can safely resume the massage. If not, you can try more of the same a little while longer. Move your hands around to different places on his body — his head, his shoulders, his own hands — and in each place follow the same pattern for several breaths, pressing lightly with his exhalation and then releasing the pressure with his inhalation. But don't expect miracles. If your friend has a serious block against permitting himself to be touched, this kind of gentle non-verbal persuasion will be unlikely to overcome it.

I might add that there are numerous other emotions which are sometimes released when the body receives a good massage. Sadness, for example; your friend may at some point find himself inadvertently crying, or wanting to cry. When you are aware of this happening be sure to interrupt the massage temporarily and encourage your friend to cry for as long as he feels like it. Usually after a few minutes of crying he will want to begin the massage again — and will probably experience the rest of the massage, in fact, as unusually calming and soothing.

Another phenomenon along these lines, one a bit more unusual, is involuntary vibrating. A sudden trembling and shaking in the flesh that can go on without stopping for some minutes, it is caused by a quick release of body energy that previously had been dammed up in constricted muscles and tissue. Usually it occurs either in the region of the stomach or the thighs, or both. Unlike the more agitated and jerky trembling that can stem from nervousness at the beginning of a massage, vibrating is a highly beneficial physical and emotional release that should be considered a part of the massage itself. Encourage your friend to let it happen, to enjoy it and not be frightened by it and to let it spread, if possible, to other parts of his body. Keep one of your hands resting against his shoulder, the back of his neck, or his head, and with the other slowly and very gently (i.e., with no pressure at all) continue to massage his body in the areas where the vibrating is taking place. Help him to keep it going — the longer it continues, the greater the release within his body. After it subsides he will feel a wonderful mixture of calm and aliveness that will most likely stay with him for several days.

Physical discomfort while a subject is lying on the massage table must be taken care of or the massage will be practically useless. Generally there are only two possible solutions: change how a subject is lying or change what he is lying on. For example, a pregnant woman (who stands to gain even more than the usual physical benefits from a massage, by the way), who cannot lie on her stomach can lie on her side while you massage her back. Or, if someone lying on his stomach feels a lot of pain in his neck when he turns it to one side, a pillow placed lengthwise under both the head and the top of the chest will permit him to turn it less, or even not at all. Other problems can be handled in similar ways — pillows can often be a great help in these matters.

And then there are the tickles, the bane of massage. Normally you will run into them when massaging the soles of the feet, sometimes also on the stomach and the sides of the torso, and occasionally in other quite unpredictable places. The one solution is heavy pressure. Press hard enough — sometimes so hard that you are one step short of causing pain to the person being massaged — and the tickles will usually evaporate. If not, then make one quick stroke over the entire area, admit defeat, and move on.

MASSAGING TO MUSIC AND OTHER EXERCISES

Three simple exercises that will add more flow and confidence to your massage touch.

First, try massing to music. I have already said that as a general rule I don't recommend playing music while you give a massage; while providing a surface pleasantness, on a deeper level it is often distracting to the person being massaged. Nevertheless, music can be an extremely valuable aid to improving your massage technique.

The idea is to make the rhythms of your strokes mesh with the rhythm of the music. Pick out a few favorite records, preferably ones having a wide variety of rhythms. Check with whomever you are going to massage to make sure that this will be okay for his or her ear, put on a record, and start in. Don't force your hands to match the music right away; just do the massage strokes that you are used to, and at the same time let yourself tune in to the music. Before long you will find your hands of their own accord trying out new patterns, and moving with a new steadiness. Be sure to experiment with other records as well. Each new rhythm will teach you some new subtlety.

Another exercise is to try "dancing" your massage. This can be done with or without accompanying music. Have your friend lie stomach down on the table — this exercise loses much of its value when done on the floor, by the way — and spread oil over the exposed surface of his body from head to feet. Then start moving your hands up and down his body. Only this time don't concentrate on him at all, nor on your own hands; instead focus entirely on the rest of your body and its movements. Enjoy yourself: dance! Move and sway all you can (keep your hands in contact, however). Experiment with as many different rhythms and patterns as you can.

It will probably surprise you to discover how greatly your entire body can become involved in the movements of massage. Also, be sure afterwards to have your friend tell you how it all felt on his side. Since you were concentrating so strongly on your own pleasure rather than on his, what he has to say may provide you with a second surprise.

One last exercise, difficult but always rewarding. Give an entire massage in complete darkness. Do everything with the sense of touch alone, including finding the oil bottle and putting on oil. You will make some mistakes and have many clumsy moments, but I can't tell you how this will help to bring your hands alive.

A variation, even more difficult: have a friend arrange for you to be led in the dark to a waiting subject that you do not know, and have never encountered before. A hard test — but one that will teach you a great deal!

No matter how much massage you may happen to know, I strongly suggest that from time to time you repeat these exercises, along with any others like them that you may happen to discover. You will always find something new in them.

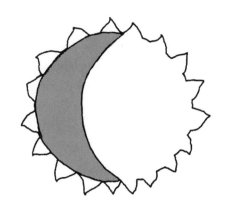

A TEN MINUTE MASSAGE

It can be done.

Not in the same way as a full massage; ten minutes is ten minutes no matter what. But if you make every minute count you can leave someone feeling surprisingly nourished.

I normally approach ten minutes of massage in one of three ways.

One is to my usual style of massage on just one or perhaps two body parts. Ten minutes of work on the back, for example; or perhaps five on the head and five more on the feet. Back, head, neck, and feet are usually the most effective places for a brief massage. If you are into trading massage with someone on a daily basis, then see to it that each part of the body gets massaged one day or another.

Another way is to cover the entire body, or close to it, by doing just one or two of your usual strokes on each part (the main stroke, for example). This method I find a bit hectic to both give and receive, but I do use it occasionally. Try it and see what you think.

A third way is to use any or all of the full-length strokes that you know on either the front or the back of the body alone, or on both. This feels superb, and is an especially good method for providing a quick energy pick-up for someone who is tired. Particularly effective are ten minutes of raking (Full-length stroke number 1) or ten minutes of working with the spread thumbs and forefingers of both hands (Full-length stroke number 5). Work on the arms as well.

And that's it. Except that the best information I have to give you in this regard is that for couples, or for anyone else sharing the same life and the same home, the ten minute massage can open the door to something extraordinary: doing massage together every day. In other words, when a day happens along on which you have the time and the inclination you trade a full massage — and on all the other days you trade ten minutes worth. I know that even ten minutes every day sounds hard; and if your life is a busy one it is hard until you get the habit of it; yet I assure you that nothing else in the world costing so little effort will as effectively change, over the course of time, the mood and tempo of your entire life. Give yourself the chance. You won't regret it.

TWO ON ONE

If you think being massaged by one person is great, wait until you try two.

Only it has to be done in the right way.

The keys to it are symmetry and tuning in. Each of the two persons doing the massage must tune in as fully to the other person doing it as to the person receiving it. Otherwise being massaged by two people feels just — well, interesting, the way maybe being massaged by an octopus would feel.

One good way to begin is with the main stroke on either the front or the back of the legs. The broad, easy sweep of this stroke will give the two of you who are doing the massage a good chance to pick up on each other's wave lengths.

You might start out by each taking one of your friend's feet, holding the foot with one hand against the sole and the other against the top of the foot. Then let your breath travel down your arms and into your hands (imagine it if you can't feel it) as you let them rest in place for a moment. Next apply the oil and begin the main stroke. Each of you can take the leg on the same side as the foot which you were holding.

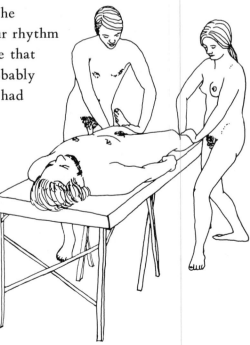

Once you have begun the main stroke, the trick of it is to match your movements and your rhythm as closely as possible. Either decide ahead of time that one of you is to lead and the other follow — probably the best way if the two of you have not already had some practice working together — or else try simply to keep your movements exactly parallel with neither of you leading, neither following.

Go up the legs at the same pace, first crossing the knees and then dividing your hands at the tops of the thighs at exactly the same moment. Try to make sure by means of any clues that you can catch hold of — (how each of you is standing, the way your hands on each side appear to press into the flesh of the leg, etc.) that you are using equal amounts of pressure. Go slow. Tune in. Your friend that you are massaging will sense exactly how much each of you is tuning in to him — and at the same time will be equally sensitive to how much the two of you are tuning in to each other.

This should give you the idea. In general it is easy to match your movements on the arms, hands, legs, and feet; just do the same massage strokes together that you are accustomed to doing singly. On the chest, stomach, buttocks and back, however, the situation is different; here, although there are a few strokes which you can do together in the same fashion (I will explain some in a moment), the rest must be done by one person working on that particular part alone. The head and neck, of course, are best left to be massaged entirely by one person.

This means you have another decision to make (again, best to make it ahead of time). During those periods where one of you is working alone somewhere around the torso or the head, the other has two options: either to stand aside and wait, or to go to work on another area at the same time even though this means that the two of you are no longer working symmetrically.

Each has its advantages. If one of you stands aside and waits, this means that your friend being massaged need suffer no confusion, that he can concentrate without distraction on what is being done to him. If, on the other hand, you decide to work somewhere else at the same time, this has the advantage of preserving the uniqueness of a double massage — your friend doesn't suddenly lose half the "touch energy" he was enjoying before.

As a rule I find that most people experience the second of these two solutions as a sensory overload and hence feel a little more comfortable with the first. There are others, however, who definitely prefer the second. You will simply have to choose for yourself, on the basis of both what the two of you feel like doing and what you feel your friend will most enjoy. One exception, by the way, to what I have just said: many people do seem to like having the head and the feet, the two poles of the body, massaged at the same time.

Fortunately there do exist a few good ways of working symmetrically, or close to it, on the front and back of the torso.

Pulling along the sides of the torso (stroke number 4 in The Back), can be done very effectively by both of you at once, both while your friend is lying on his back and while he

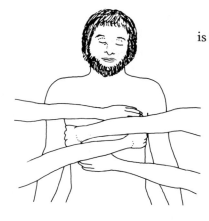

is lying on his stomach. Stand on opposite sides of the table and reach across to the side of your friend's torso which is away from you. Have one of your arm's between your partner's arms, and keep all four arms close together — touching or almost touching. Keep your strokes slow and steady, and make sure they are evenly matched.

Another superb stroke: one of you must stand at the head end of the table and do the main stroke on either the front or the back of the torso (stroke number 1 in The Chest and Stomach; stroke number 1 in The Back). The other stands at the foot end of the table and does the main stroke on both legs at once (as in stroke 6 in Full-length Strokes, without, however, going onto the back). The idea is to make all four hands move in the same direction at the same time. This means that one of you must wait and then begin just as the other is completing the first half of his stroke. In other words, while one pair of hands is heading up the sides of the torso toward the shoulders, the other pair heads up the legs toward the hips; and vice versa.

Another stroke for the back and the buttocks: the Giant Hand. Lock all four hands together by entwining your fingers as shown in the illustration. This will create a sort of oversized hand which the two of you can then make flow back and forth in every direction. Feels very good.

A number of the other full-length strokes described in the instruction sections can be done by two persons at once. Try raking; try the main stroke up one leg and then all the way up the back; try the bear walk; try long strokes with the stretched thumb and forefinger of one hand; try feather-light strokes.

Finally, letting all four hands "roam" with no symmetry and no apparent pattern for a short period of time can be an excellent way to end a double massage.

As I have said, many subjects will feel uncomfortable, as if split several ways at once, if you try this early in the massage. Coming later, however, it will feel much better. For one reason, your friend's body will now be more relaxed and open; for another, the strangeness of being touched by two people at the same time will have passed.

Do double massage from time to time. Besides being fun to do, it will leave you more versatile at massage in general. Double massage is a little like doing massage to music: tuning in to a partner's massage rhythm teaches you new possibilities for your own.

One last comment: doing double massage for a friend can be an especially fine experience for a couple. The act of mutually caring for a third person, plus the sensitivity to each other demanded at the same time, create a space in which a couple can experience their own closeness in a new and powerful way.

SELF-MASSAGE

Being your own masseur is a little like being your own lover. It can be done, but somehow it just isn't the same thing.

There are several problems. Most obvious, I suppose, is that there are some areas of your body which you cannot reach. And others which you can, but not with the right dexterity and leverage.

This is actually the least of the difficulties, however. More important is that you can't fully relax. No one part of your body can completely relax while another part is busy at work; the body is too closely interconnected for that.

Also, your attention is split. When doing massage your attention must be on the activity of your hands; when receiving it you need to concentrate on letting go, on allowing yourself to be taken care of. Trying to do both at once means that you can really give yourself up to neither, and the massage done in this way can't help but remain superficial.

Most crucial of all, however, is that no communication and no exchange of energy can take place when you do massage on yourself. The expressive side of massage falls away, and what is left is something completely mechanical; a physical technique and nothing more.

Having said all this, let me now add what I think self-massage is in fact good for. First of all, if you are feeling tired and numb it can sometimes help bring your body awake. Second, a healthy physical relationship with yourself of this kind has its own psychological rewards. Learning to touch your own body is a good means of learning to accept it. Finally — and this is where, for anyone into massage, the real value of self-massage lies — it can show you a great deal about what feels good and what doesn't in massage. It can teach you about the hidden architecture of bone and muscle, about the effects of greater and lesser amounts of pressure, and much more. You can use it as a valuable kind of exploration and feedback. The more you know about your own body, the more you will know about everyone else's.

I find that the best techniques for self-massage are kneading and squeezing, hard pressure with the fingertips, and slapping. Oil is not necessary. In fact it is next to useless; the type of strokes that require it cannot be done in self-massage because of insufficient leverage.

There is not a great deal that you need to be told in terms of specific directions. Simply press, poke and squeeze wherever you can — experiment and explore. Here are a few things which you might try.

Face and scalp. Work either lying on your back or sitting up. On your back is a little better for your face, sitting up a little better for your scalp. For the face you can do most of what you do when massaging someone else; use your fingertips instead of your thumbs on the forehead, however. For the scalp, lots of vigorous rubbing with the fingertips.

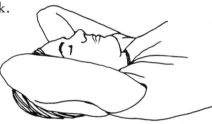

Neck and upper back (1). Lie on your back. Press as hard as you can with your fingertips just to either side of the spine; wiggle your fingertips in place a little as you press. Start just below the spine as far under the back as you can reach. (You will probably not get much farther than a point about parallel with the tops of the shoulder blades.) Then do the same thing just above the shoulder blades, working from the spine outwards to the shoulders.

Neck and upper back (2). Sit in a chair. First let your head (but only your head) hang as far forward as possible. Then, pressing hard with your fingertips, make tiny circles just below the base of the skull; work from about two inches to one side of the spine to about two inches to the other side. Next, with your head again upright, let one arm and shoulder go as limp as possible. With the fingertips of the opposite hand press hard just above the top of the shoulder blade; move your fingertips slightly as you press. Go slowly all the way across the top of the blade, starting at the shoulder and working towards the spine. Then go down the side of the blade closest to the spine as far as you can reach (it won't be very far).

Chest. Knead and press with the fingertips while either sitting up or lying down.

Stomach. Rub in a circle with one palm. Then gently press and knead with the fingertips.

Sides of the torso. Knead and rub.

Lower and middle back. This one is hard. Animals that rub against tree trunks probably have the best idea. The only effective thing I know to do is to stand and to press the tips of your thumbs as hard as you can just to either side of your spine. Start an inch or two above the base of the spine; press each time for about five seconds and then move your thumbs up a half an inch or so and press again. Work your way up as high onto the middle back as you can reach.

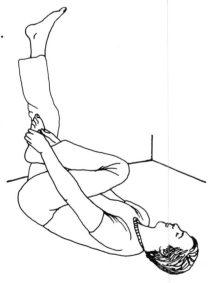

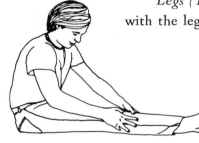

Legs (1). Sit on the ground or on a bed with the legs extended. Knead and press with the fingertips.

Legs (2). Lie on your back with your legs propped up against a wall or a piece of furniture. Lower one foot so that it is just within reach. Working down-ward from the foot, knead and squeeze the foot and the entire leg. Repeat as many times as you like, working downward only. (This helps the veins to drain toward the heart.)

Buttocks. Knead, either while standing or while lying on your stomach.

Feet. Here you can do your best work, especially on the sole of the foot. Sit in a chair and rest one foot on the opposite thigh. At this angle you can work carefully and with plenty of pressure over the entire sole. Then with your fingers and thumbs work the rest of the foot. Don't forget the toes.

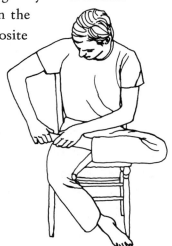

Everywhere. Slap! Slap every square inch of the body that you can reach. Include the face, slapping more lightly. I find this more fun — and quicker — than any other form of self-massage.

So there you are. Let me add one more comment. To my mind, the real singular or one-person equivalent of massage is not self-massage, but hatha yoga. If, despite my discouraging remarks, you find that self-massage does something magical for you, then you might explore whether yoga may not be able to do the same and much more.

YOUR ANIMALS TOO

By all means massage your animals. They will love it, and you will learn a few things. Born connoisseurs of massage, animals give feedback of an unmatched eloquence. Do the right thing and they will sprawl in a heap on the floor. Do the wrong thing and they will snap at you or paw your hands away.

The main rule when doing animal massage is to explore the bone structure. Here is an anatomical structure foreign to what you are used to working on; find out how it works, what its underlying shape is, and how you can adapt to it any of the massage techniques you are familiar with.

A few tips.

Pay particular attention to an animal's spine. Working up and down in the two furrows lying just to either side of the spine is almost always effective.

Don't neglect the base of the skull, an equally responsive place. It must be as high a tension area for animals as it is for humans, judging from the way they react to its being massaged.

Probe all around the shoulder blades. You can often go in quite deep between the blades and the spine. Always press gently at first, but don't be afraid gradually to try harder pressure. If an animal senses that you have just the right place, he will usually let you press surprisingly hard.

Individual animals seem to vary greatly when it comes to the stomach. Some don't want it touched at all. Others love having their stomachs lightly kneaded.

In general try to keep your touch consistently focused and definite. Animals tune in almost immediately, and if they feel that you know what you are doing they will start trusting you right away.

I'm pretty much a dog and cat man myself. I've never really gotten into horses and buffaloes, or for that matter mice and canaries, all of which I'm sure are whole massage worlds unto themselves.

No species is an island.

MASSAGE FOR LOVERS

Bet you turned to this chapter right away, huh?

In that case, unless you are already well acquainted with massage, you may find it difficult to believe the first thing I have here to say: ordinary massage and erotic massage are two separate kinds of experience, and they lie many miles apart. The more massage you do and receive, the more you will come to appreciate this difference. One is sensual, the other sexual. One leaves the body feeling calm, the other leaves it feeling aroused.

Between your mate or lover and yourself an exchange of ordinary massage will always be a beautiful thing. For a couple, however, massage obviously offers other directions as well. To a greater degree than anything else I know of, massage can make sex both physically and psychologically more fulfilling. For a couple having difficulties with sexual intimacy, for example, it can add that critical element of mutual trust and relaxation which formerly was lacking from their physical relationship; I have known many couples who have made this discovery. And for the couple between whom sex is already mutually satisfying, massage can provide the means to an increased richness difficult to describe.

The key to erotic massage is not, as you might expect, a detailed massaging of the genitals. Naturally this can feel exquisite, and in itself it is fine as a part of sexual massage — but only as a part. The main focus of sexual massage should be something slightly different: the energizing and eroticization of the entire body. This experience alone can add to sex something completely new in quality, something more than a heightened intensity.

But how? The answer is that an erotic massage must proceed by stages. The boundaries between these stages hardly need to be exact, and they certainly don't have to be done in the order mentioned here. The important thing is merely that each stage be included, and that each receive its share of unhurried attention.

The first is simply that of ordinary massage. Give your partner a complete body massage of the kind described earlier in this book. Be as brief as you want, but make sure that every part of the body is thoroughly covered.

Next do feather-light stroking with the fingertips all over the body. I have already suggested that at the end of an ordinary massage you do a little of this (Full-length stroke number 6). For erotic massage, however, do much more; ten, twenty, any number of times more. This will greatly heighten the sexual sensitivity of your partner's body throughout its entire length. You don't even need to wait until you have finished the period of ordinary massage; you can include soft stroking at the same time, gradually increasing the amount as you go.

The next step is to concentrate more fully on those areas of the body which, other than and in addition to the genitals, carry a heightened sexual charge. These include primarily the pelvic region and the regions immediately joining — the stomach, the insides of the thighs, the buttocks, and the lower back — and the breasts. But also give some attention to the ears, the lips, the back of the neck, the palms, the insides of the elbows, the armpits, the soles of the feet, the big toe, and the backs of the knees — all areas which respond easily to sexual vibrations. Do some additional ordinary massage work on these areas, returning to soft stroking whenever you wish.

Next comes the most important stage of all: connecting the genitals with the rest of the body. Here the idea is to do strokes which at some point lightly touch or graze the genitals, and which from there go immediately to others parts of the body. The effect this will have, especially coming after a period of full body soft stroking, will be to gradually transfer some of the higher sexual excitation usually associated with the genitals to the rest of the body as well.

The final stage is of course to focus your attention on your partner's genitals themselves. Pressing lightly with your fingertips, work slowly and with great care over the entire genital region. Cover each surface with tiny circles, outline the contours of each distinct part with one fingertip, and the like. Concentrate not on arousing your partner — this will happen by itself — but on making him or her feel that his or her genitals are a part of the body on a par with other parts, worthy of the same kind of attention and nuturing care.

What strokes and techniques should you use for erotic massage? For the most part you will find it easy to adapt those which you have already learned for ordinary massage. Just follow your own instincts and intuitions; when it comes to doing erotic massage with someone you love, the imagination is the most important organ which you have. Here are a few specific suggestions. (Note: much of this will probably make little sense unless you have already become familiar with the instruction section of this book.)

➴ When doing feather-light stroking, move your hands so that your fingertips are barely brushing against your partner's skin. Work up and down the entire length of his or her body. Go sometimes slowly and sometimes a little faster; sometimes in straight lines and sometimes in waves, circles, spirals, or whatever.

🪝 A good variation of feather-light stroking: use just the tip of one finger of one hand. Move it slowly all around the body. Though this looks more or less the same as using your entire hand, your partner will experience it as something distinctly different.

🪝 Here is a good additional stroke for either a man's or a woman's chest. Place the tips of both thumbs immediately next to and on opposite sides of one nipple. Pressing lightly, draw both thumb tips at the same time (but moving in opposite directions) directly outwards. Stop when you have reached the outer edges of the breast on a woman, or when the thumbs are about five inches apart on a man. Then return the thumbs to the nipple and, as if you were drawing the spokes of a wheel, do the same thing starting at points a fraction of an inch or so farther around. Continue in the same way, taking a total of about eight simultaneous strokes with both thumb tips to cover the entire breast.

🪝 For the feet: run one finger slowly all the way in and out between each pair of toes.

🪝 Try reversing your hands when doing the main stroke on the back of the leg — i.e., lead with your right hand instead of your left while massaging the left leg. Take both hands right over the top of the buttock before dividing them; then, as you take your outside hand (the left in this example) over the hip as usual, glide your inside hand lightly down between the buttocks and over any part of the genitals easily within reach before heading both hands back down the leg.

🪝 Work the fingertips of one hand in tiny circles around the tip of the coccyx (the tail bone). Use firm pressure, concentrating on the surrounding muscles rather than the bone itself. Then work more lightly down to the genitals and back, and then again more firmly around the coccyx.

🪝 Leading with the heel of the hand, bring one hand in a single steady motion up from the genitals, between the buttocks, up the spine and, turning the hand sideways now, onto the back of the neck. Let this hand rest on the back of the neck and repeat the same thing with the other hand; take the first away a little before you reach the neck with the second. Continue like this, alternating hands each time and having one hand always resting against the back of the neck while the other is moving.

✎ Make tiny circles with the fingertips of one hand up and down the groove between the pelvis and the inside of the thigh on each side. Work slowly, and use plenty of pressure. Go several times all the way up and down on each side. Then, much more lightly, go briefly onto the genitals. Then, pressing the same as before, again between the pelvis and the thigh.

✎ Move the tip of one forefinger in a tiny circle at the center of the top of your partner's head. Move the tip of the other forefinger in a tiny circle on the perineum — a spot about the size of a coin between the rectum and the genitals. Press moderately. Keep both fingers moving slowly in unison for a minute or longer.

✎ For the vagina itself, try placing the tips of both thumbs on the perineum (c.f. the previous stroke) with one thumb tip directly above the other. Pressing lightly, move both thumb tips together straight upwards to the top of the vaginal inner lips. Then separate the thumbs, one going to the right and one to the left; pressing more firmly, bring them down between the inner and the outer lips all the way to the perineum. Continue the same circular movement without stopping.

✎ For the penis, place the tips of both forefingers against the perineum. Separate the forefingers, moving one to the right and one to the left, and follow the edges of the scrotum to the base of the penis. Continue without a break directly onto the penis, bringing the tips of the forefingers together again at the base of the underside (the side that is exposed when the penis is erect). Glide both forefingers together straight up the length of the penis, going over and down to the opposite side of the head. Then, pressing just below the lower ridge of the head (the coronal ridge), separate the fingers again and, following the ridge around, bring them both back onto the underside of the penis. Then, with the fingertips once more together, go back down the penis and around the scrotum all the way back to the perineum. Repeat without stopping.

Go on from here however you wish. Without hurry!

One last suggestion for couples. Do erotic massage together whenever you feel like it, but try if you have time to share frequent sessions of ordinary massage as well. In other words, try to expand your relationship within the world of touch in as many directions as possible. I guarantee that this will help to enrich your relationship in other dimensions as well.

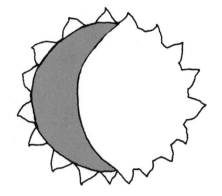

GETTING DEEPER INTO IT: SOME DIRECTIONS

Perhaps by now you have mastered most of the strokes listed in the instruction section of this book. Perhaps you have also gone on, as was suggested in some later chapters, to explore other ways of using these techniques, and have had the satisfaction of seeing emerge from your experiments the beginnings of a massage style uniquely your own.

If so, you may feel that you have learned enough. And in a sense I could only agree with you. Give yourself a bit more practice along the same lines, and you will soon be doing massage as well as the average professional masseur or masseuse.

Perhaps, however, despite having come this far, you feel that you are not yet prepared to stop; that massage still holds something more for you, something deeper. In that case you are ready for the next step.

From this point on, getting deeper into massage means, in my opinion, that you must follow a single road: that of getting deeper into your own body.

Wherever in this book I have spoken of doing massage with your hands, this has been a convenient fiction. Massage is done (whether well or poorly) with the entire body; with its particular style, its gestures, and its degree of aliveness; with the living sum of all one's attitudes towards and about it.

Nevertheless most of us are, in actual fact, largely cut off from the body; ordinarily we are in contact with only a fraction of its inner richness. And it is exactly about this that you must do something. Change the manner and degree to which you are aware of your own body, and you will radically change the way you do massage — and much else besides! Far more than we tend to realize, the very feel and texture of our lives is shaped by the way we live and experience our bodies. For myself, I know that many of the things that have made my massage better have made my life better as well.

How does one go about increasing his awareness of his own body? There are many ways, fortunately. I have mine; you will have yours. What I want to share with you here are some hints which, I feel, have a particular relevance to massage.

Let's look first at a few ideas about the body. Take them on a purely intellectual level, and, far from helping, they will only get in your way. Take them, however, as signposts for feeling, as ideas to be lived — and you may discover in them a key to many things within yourself.

    You are your body. Today this is a truism in much of psychology and philosophy; another familiar way of putting it is that mind and body are one and the same. Our emotions, our outer perceptions, our spiritual life, and even our conceptual understanding of the world around us all begin and end within this intimate shadowy mass which is our being. Our body, its possibilities of movement, and its relation to gravity and the earth are the background from which everything else must emerge. To come to terms with this on a real emotional level is perhaps the most important kind of self-encounter a person can have. As Alexander Lowen puts it: "When the ego roots itself in the body, an individual gains insight into himself. The deeper the roots, the deeper the insight."

    Yet, consciously or unconsciously, we tend still to resist the notion that we literally are our bodies. The ideas and suggestions that follow, while dependent upon this primary idea, perhaps at the same time can offer a means of coming more to grips with it.

    The sense of touch is as important a contact with reality as the sense of sight. For centuries in our Western culture we have allowed the world as encountered by sight almost totally to dominate the world as encountered by touch. Learning to live again in the world of touch is for us now like travelling to a new and very strange country.

    The place to begin is not just at the massage table, but also during the course of your daily life. Learn to dwell on the weight and texture of an object you pick up; on the feel and balance of your body where it presses against the chair you sit in, or the ground you walk on; on whatever you feel happening each time your body and the world make contact. Learn also to respond with your entire body, letting the feel of an object in your fingers, or of the sole of your foot against the floor, echo and reverberate everywhere within you.

    Two books with a number of practical exercises that can help you to explore your sense of touch are Bernard Gunther's *Sense Relaxation Below Your Mind* (Collier), and Frederick Perls, Ralph F. Hefferline, and Paul Goodman's *Gestalt Therapy* (Delta).

    Be patient, and respect the newness of what you are trying to do. Imagine yourself as a being from another planet trying to enjoy the realities of this one through a sense-form that you have never had to use before.

✍ *Your body tends constantly to express itself.* It does so in many different ways and on many different levels.

Probably no other discovery has had a greater impact upon the human potential movement. Because we reveal through gesture, posture and movement so much more than we are fully aware of, the practice of "reading" body language — unfolding the body's non-verbal messages and translating them into words — has become an important tool in gestalt therapy and the gestalt-oriented encounter group. (Take a look, for example, at Fritz Perls's highly readable *Gestalt Therapy Verbatim* (Real People Press) and at Williams Schutz's *Here Comes Everybody* (Harper and Row).

What this means for massage is, I think, that the quality of one's touch has an expressive range far wider than has ordinarily been thought to be the case. The body is permeated with a communicative force; and touching, no less than any other of its activities, takes place constantly within the field of this force.

Learn to "listen" to your sense of touch (at all times, not just while doing massage) much the way you might listen to the sound of your own voice. Accept that you express yourself through touch — that in fact you can't help expressing yourself so — and tune in all you can to the ways in which you do so.

Even the objects in your hands or that your body otherwise comes into contact with — imagine yourself as greeting them, questioning them, talking to them through touch. Something like this does seem to happen on a primitive level, and with patience you can tune in to it. Learn to recognize your body as a flow of expressive interaction with both people and objects; as a web of mute speech endlessly being spun between yourself and the world.

✍ *Your body is a field of energy.* Different traditions have called this energy by different names. In yoga it is the "prana." In Tai Chi Chaun, a form of moving meditation developed in China, it is the "chi;" in Aikido, a Japanese form of awareness and self-defense, the "ki." Wilhelm Reich, coming to the same thing by a very different path, called it "bio-electrical" and "orgone" energy. Today most of the human potential movement, including Reich's most direct successors in bioenergetic therapy, has settled simply for "energy."

Although unalike in their methods, these different approaches have certain basic ideas in common about the nature and meaning of body energy. Central to all of them is the conviction that this energy can be directly experienced, that the whole point of becoming more deeply aware of the body is in fact to experience it and that many of the higher stages of personal growth are inseparable from increasingly enriched experiences of this sort.

What can the physicist, the chemist, and the biologist tell us about the nature of this energy? So far, next to nothing. From a scientific point of view this energy has yet to be "seen." That is, no instrument has yet been found which can effectively locate and measure it. A small amount of research has been undertaken (e.g., bio-feedback experiments in this country, acupuncture research in France and Russia), but its results are of a highly tentative and preliminary nature.

This means that we are dealing with a scientific unknown. Even the language used to describe it is highly metaphorical and vague. And yet there is no question that this energy — this "something" — can be felt from within. For centuries men have been charting some of its inward patterns and exploring ways to increase its flow. Anyone can be taught to feel it, to heighten it, to experience it more intensely and more subtly. And, I might add, beyond a certain point there is nothing else I know of that will so enrich your awareness of your body.

Here as before there is much that you can do by yourself. The main thing is, whenever you tune in to your body, to think of yourself not as a "thing," but as a field of energy capable of experiencing its own inner dynamics. However, don't try to predict too closely what this will feel like, or what it would feel like if you were doing it "correctly." Just tune in, playing at the same time with the notions of 'energy' and 'field,' and see what happens.

A few additional clues: one good way to start is to take frequent notice of what parts of your body seem most alive; and what parts seem least alive, or seem even not to be present.

Remember also that as a field of energy your body is a process; it is always in a state of flux. Pay careful attention to the aliveness or deadness of a single part, for example, and you will see that it never stays the same. Be aware also of any sensations of inner flow, warmth or tingling. The more subtle your attention, the greater number of minute changes you will experience taking place.

Whenever you have difficulty getting in touch with your body energy there are two devices that will almost always help. One is to focus on your breath. Follow its rhythm, its changes and fluctuations, and the smoothness or jerkiness of its rise and fall; stay alert both to the breath itself and to any muscular movements or sensations accompanying it elsewhere in the body. The other is called "centering." The center of your body is your abdomen; it is what in Japanese culture is called the *hara*. To center yourself is to focus your attention on the central region of your abdomen and to let whatever you are doing — actions, feelings, seeing, speaking — unfold itself from this point. Focusing on the breath, and centering, can also be very effectively combined:

follow the movement of your breath as before, but let each inhalation sink straight to the center of your abdomen. Even better: imagine that your breath, passing through and on all sides around this center point, is with each inhalation filling your entire body.

If you would like to try a small exercise that can help you to experience your breath in this manner, here is one of many developed by Magda Proskauer. Lie on your back. Let your body relax as fully as you can. Then with your breath do the following: (1) Begin inhaling through the nose and exhaling out the mouth. (2) Let your breath become as quiet, as smooth and as long as it wants to be without, however, forcing it in any manner. (3) After each exhalation see if you can allow a pause to take place before inhaling again. Don't, however, do anything to actively "hold" the breath out. Instead just don't do anything at all to bring it back in — in other words, let yourself wait until the breath comes back entirely of its own accord. (Don't worry, it will always come back!) (4) Let each breath go straight to the abdomen. Don't worry about using the chest at all. Explore how much space you can feel within your abdomen, and to what extent you can feel each inhalation filling that space.

Next, if you would like to take this exercise a step further, add the following. (1) Continue with the same breathing pattern — in the nose and out the mouth, pausing after the exhalation, and letting each inhalation go all the way to the abdomen. (2) On every alternate breath, gently tighten your right buttock as you inhale. Make the movement as smooth as possible. Try to isolate the buttock muscles so that you are not flexing the muscles anywhere else in your body. At the same time send your inhalation right into the buttock itself. (3) Release the buttock as you exhale, letting the buttock settle into the floor as much as it wants to go. Make this movement also as smooth as possible. At the same time imagine that your exhalation is going right out the buttock itself. (4) Continue these two movements on every other breath. Rest, without moving, on the in between breaths. (5) After several minutes move to your left buttock and repeat. (6) After doing the same on both sides, again let your breath simply filter down towards your abdomen, and see what sense of inner space you now can feel in this portion of your body.

One last general clue: don't fall into the trap of trying to separate "physical sensations" from "emotional qualities." To tune in to the energy which is your body is to feel neither just the one nor just the other, but the common root of both.

You don't have to stop here, however. By experimenting with the way of thinking and the activities suggested above you can learn many things. Nevertheless this represents only a beginning. As already mentioned, there are a number of more structured methods of heightening the awareness of one's own body. Some are Eastern disciplines having long traditions: meditation, yoga, Tai Chi Chaun and Aikido are several currently most popular. Others are more recent Western developments: for example, Proskauer breath techniques (a highly simplified example of which was just given above), group work in sensory awareness, and bioenergetic therapy.

If you want to develop as much skill and presence as possible in the practice of massage, I strongly recommend that you explore one or more of these approaches. Whichever you choose to try out, the very fact of your having some familiarity with massage will give you a head start. Among the various forms of "body work" there is a great deal of overlap, and the practice of one tends strongly to reinforce the practice of any others.

You will discover for yourself which is most suited to your needs. All are of immense value in themselves, and all are helpful for massage as well.

However, among these various approaches there are two which, I am convinced, are especially valuable for massage: meditation and Tai Chi Chaun. I would like to say a little more about these in the next two chapters.

MEDITATION

Like massage, meditation is done with the entire body.

This is not always explicitly recognized. The directions given the student of meditation usually emphasize what not to do: don't pursue thoughts; don't leave the present moment; don't move your body, etc. And this is only right, for the initial purpose of all meditation is to bring a temporary stop to the buzz and drone of our verbal thinking.

But what happens once our internal verbal chatter begins to quiet down? The answer is that eventually a lot happens; specifically what depending in part on the particular type of meditation being practiced. Whatever the type, however, one of the most important effects will be a highly intensified awareness of the body. Internal verbal chatter is a defense against feeling the body. Remove some of this defense, and the field of energy that is the body can't help but make itself felt more strongly.

Whatever else happens — depending, as I have said, upon the particular type of meditation — is a development of this intensified body awareness. Once meditation is taken to a certain depth the body becomes like a rich music that can be played in any of a great variety of ways. There are some forms of meditation, for example, which lead simply to a sense of calmness and inner harmony; this calmness, however, remains thoroughly a physical one, a serenity that seeps through the body almost like a physical warmth. Other types explicitly make use of a focusing of attention on a single part of the body: for example, the abdomen or *hara,* or the "third eye" center in the forehead. A few of these latter types offer, if pursued far enough, what their practictioners feel is the most intense experience known to man: a sensation of one's body energy becoming fused with the vaster energies of the cosmos.

Whatever the type of meditation practiced, for anyone into massage the side benefits are enormous. Make meditation a daily habit for a period of some months or more, and you will find yourself bringing to the massage table a sensitivity and inner focus which you would never have thought possible.

How can you learn? The best way is to find a good teacher. However, if the right teacher — right for you, no matter what he may seem to be for others — doesn't appear to be available, I would suggest exploring a few good books. Two helpful overviews of the different forms of meditation are Christmas Humphreys, *Concentration And Meditation* (Shambala), and Claudio Naranjo and Robert E. Ornstein, *On The Psychology Of Meditation* (Viking).

A beautiful work on Zen meditation, invaluable for anyone beginning meditation whether he is specifically interested in Zen or not, is Yasutani's lectures in Philip Kapleau, ed., *Three Pillars Of Zen* (Beacon).

Another fine book on Zen meditation is Shunryo Suzuki's *Zen Mind, Beginner's Mind* (Weatherhill).

Which kind should you try? This depends strictly on you, and what fits for you. There are any number of ways from which to pick. Depending on which you choose, for example, you may be instructed to keep your eyes open or closed; to breathe naturally or in a specific rhythm; to let your mind stay visually "blank" or to concentrate on certain images; silently to repeat to yourself a word or phrase called a mantra, or to keep yourself from verbally concentrating on anything at all." My suggestion is that you experiment all you can. The important thing is to get started, and any style of meditation that helps you do that is for you a good style.

Any style is also excellent for massage. However, at this point I will share with you one piece of admittedly prejudiced advice. For reasons which I will explain in a later chapter, I think that any form of meditation which includes both some kind of active dwelling upon the breath, and some amount of concentration on the abdomen or *hara*, will have a few unique extra benefits for the practice of massage.

Zazen, for example, a style of meditation associated with the Eastern Zen tradition, includes both of these. So do some Yoga meditations which include focusing upon energy centers (usually called *chakras*) in the lower as well as the upper parts of the body. And there are others.

Here is a simple meditation with which you might experiment. It includes elements of both yoga and Zen traditions. (1) Sit with your back comfortably straight. Sit cross-legged on a small firm cushion if you can do so without straining; if not, sit in a straight-backed chair with your knees a couple of feet apart. (2) Breathe through the nose. Don't do anything to your breath, and don't change its rhythm in any way — with one exception. Do let yourself pause after each exhalation; try completely to suspend all activity on your part, and to let the breath come back in entirely of its own accord (i.e., the same as for the Proskauer breath exercise given at the end of the previous chapter). (4) Also let each breath sink as low as you can and let it go into your abdomen. Don't force it to move lower; just be sure to let it go as low as it wants to go. (5) Count your breaths. Count on each exhaltion, going from one to ten and then start again at one. Repeat the same pattern for as long as you meditate. (6) For the first five minutes or so focus all your attention on the center of your abdomen, however vaguely or sharply you may feel yourself to be in touch with that center. Then for the remainder of the period of meditation focus your attention at the middle of the forehead, on a point about half an inch above the bridge of the nose and about half an inch inside. (7) Don't pursue thoughts. Try to let your mind become empty and still. Give all your attention to whichever point of the body you are concentrating on, and to the feel and flow of your breath. (8) Give up all expectations. Try to be content with whatever happens, even if for some time this means nothing at all. (9) Don't try to meditate too long in the beginning. Ten minutes a day is fine. Gradually increase this amount when you feel ready. Begin each time by focusing for five minutes or so at the center of the abdomen, and then move your attention to the middle of the forehead.

In general I find that, once a certain familiarity with the techniques and effects of meditation has been attained, elements of practice taken from different traditions can be very effectively combined. Say, for example, you have found a meditation that suits you well, but which does not include either centering (focusing on the abdomen) or dwelling upon the breath. You might then try either in some way combining these elements with your meditation itself (I would try this only if you have become fairly advanced in your practice), or else adding them during a short preliminary period at the beginning of your regular sitting. In short, experiment — it pays off.

TAI CHI CHUAN

If the gods themselves were to give us something to make massage better, I suspect it would look a lot like Tai Chi Chuan. I am told that among the Chinese, who consider massage a high art, it is common for a masseur to take up the practice of Tai Chi as an integral part of his massage training. The reasons are not hard to understand.

Tai Chi is a form of moving meditation developed in China some generations ago. Based both upon the movements of animals and many traditional fighting movements, it consists of a series of slow, dance-like steps and gestures of the entire body. Depending on the particular school and the speed with which it's done, Tai Chi takes from about five to thirty minutes to perform, or, as the Chinese say, to "play." Although extremely beautiful from the point of view of the outside observer, the essence of Tai Chi lies not in its visual qualities but in the feel of it on the inside for the person who does it.

What makes it so fine for massage? Most obvious is the flowing quality of the movements of the hands. When doing Tai Chi the hands look like fish moving slowly through water. Yet every movement is absolutely precise and, despite its graceful-ness, often performed with a great deal of hidden strength. This combination of smoothness and pre-cision is also exactly what our hands need to acquire for doing massage.

Equally important for massage are the stance and the movements of the rest of the body. Minute attention is given to balance and gravity, to centering, and to the exact movements, internal and external, of the torso and legs in order to provide a base for the flowing gestures of the hands.

Finally, for the advanced student Tai Chi is unquestionably a form of meditation. Concentration is focused on the abdomen, attention is given to the breath, and energy is made to circulate

142

throughout the body. As we will point out in more detail in the next chapter, these are inward activities which can be used with great benefit at the massage table as well.

I wish I could tell you an easy way to learn Tai Chi Chuan. Unfortunately, a trained instructor is necessary — without one you don't stand a chance of learning it correctly — and at the present moment decent teachers are few and far between. Two prominent in this country are Li Li-Ta in San Francisco and Chang Man Cheng in New York. Teachers also can occasionally be found at growth centers, free universities, and in other cities having a large Chinese community.

This situation is improving, however, and in the near future will no doubt improve even more. Wherever Tai Chi today is available, it is becoming immensely popular. Within a few years we will very likely see a new generation of teachers, and a far greater number of them, offering instruction in Tai Chi in many different parts of this country.

In the meantime all I can say is that if you are into massage, and if you ever do have the chance to learn some Tai Chi Chuan, take it. At least give it a try. Watch it being done, experiment with a few of the beginning movements, and see if Tai Chi speaks to you. If it does, I assure you that you are on your way to learning a lot more about massage.

THE NEXT STEP

Energy, meditation, Tai Chi, the body as self . . . what do they all mean when it comes time to actually give a friend a massage?

Largely a change of orientation. Up to this point while doing massage you most likely have been concentrating entirely on your friend and his or her needs. In itself this is good; certainly it is the fastest way to learn massage. The next step, however, is to learn to tune in to yourself at the same time. And this means, of course, tuning in to your body; into its mood and feel, its balance, its energy.

This is not an easy switch. In the beginning you will probably find it awkward. For a period of time, in fact, tuning in to yourself may even interfere with your ability to focus your attention on your friend. Don't worry, however; the change will come. And the more you let yourself follow a few of the paths suggested in the previous chapters, the faster it will come.

Also, don't let yourself be fooled by a false notion of the economics of attention. It's not true that you have only a fixed "amount" of attention; giving some to yourself doesn't mean that you have to give less to your friend. At first it may well feel that way. Before long, however, you will find that your own body, more resonant and feeling within, will have become a better receiver of what lies without and that, far from giving your friend less attention, by tuning in to yourself you can give him more.

Beyond this there is not a great deal I can tell you; or need to. The following hints, however, may help you to get started.

✍ Stay as much as you can in the present moment. Let outside thoughts distract you as little as possible. If you have undertaken meditation as a regular practice, try to be present to yourself now with the same fullness.

✍ Stay aware of your breathing. While doing massage breathe always through the nose. Follow your breath; let it go as low as it can into your body, and, without forcing it in any way, let it become as long and smooth as possible.

✍ Focus on the center of your body — the internal center of your abdomen or *hara*, however and wherever you feel it. Send your breath to this point if that helps you to stay aware of it. Think of yourself as doing massage from this place. Feel it as a source, a depth from which everything done with your hands can naturally emerge.

↩ Don't program too rigidly what you intend to do during a massage. Keep yourself fresh. Be clear about the order you want to use for working on the different parts of the body, also about what parts, if any, you suspect may require special attention. Beyond that, however, (assuming that you by now are familiar with a sufficient amount of technique) rely upon your spontaneity and your sensitivity to what your hands are feeling rather than a detailed plan of action worked out in advance.

↩ Be aware of the ground beneath you. Sense the floor beneath your feet, sense the support of the massage table as you gently press your friend against it, and sense your own balance between these points. Think of yourself as exploring with your friend his and your mutual connection with this supporting ground.

↩ Be as alert as you can to the flow of energy in your own body. Try — in any way that feels natural, whether imagined or felt — to send energy to your friend with your hands, just as a healer does.

↩ At the same time try to tune in to the flow of energy within your friend's body. This is extremely difficult at first, but with practice you will be surprised at how much your hands will be able to tell you. Don't have any preconceptions about what this will or won't feel like. Just tune in, and see what happens.

↩ Remember that massage is always a form of non-verbal communication — but remember as well that the body tends naturally to express itself. This means that the communicative side of massage is not something external, something added; instead it is something already present and what we have to learn is how not to interfere with it. Massage is not Morse code: you don't need to worry about having a "message" in mind before you begin.

Perhaps an analogy will help. Gestalt therapists often comment that the sound and the vocal mannerisms of a person's voice express far more than the actual content of what he is saying. The same applies to massage: although many attitudes and signals can be easily translated by using the hands, it is the quality itself of a person's touch which offers the greatest range of expression.

In other words, trust the body; let yourself be as fully rooted and present within it as possible; and communication will take care of itself.

In sum, massage is an act of celebration, an act in which the experience of the giver is as important as the experience of the receiver. Approach it as such, and you will learn from within yourself everything else about it which you might ever want to know.

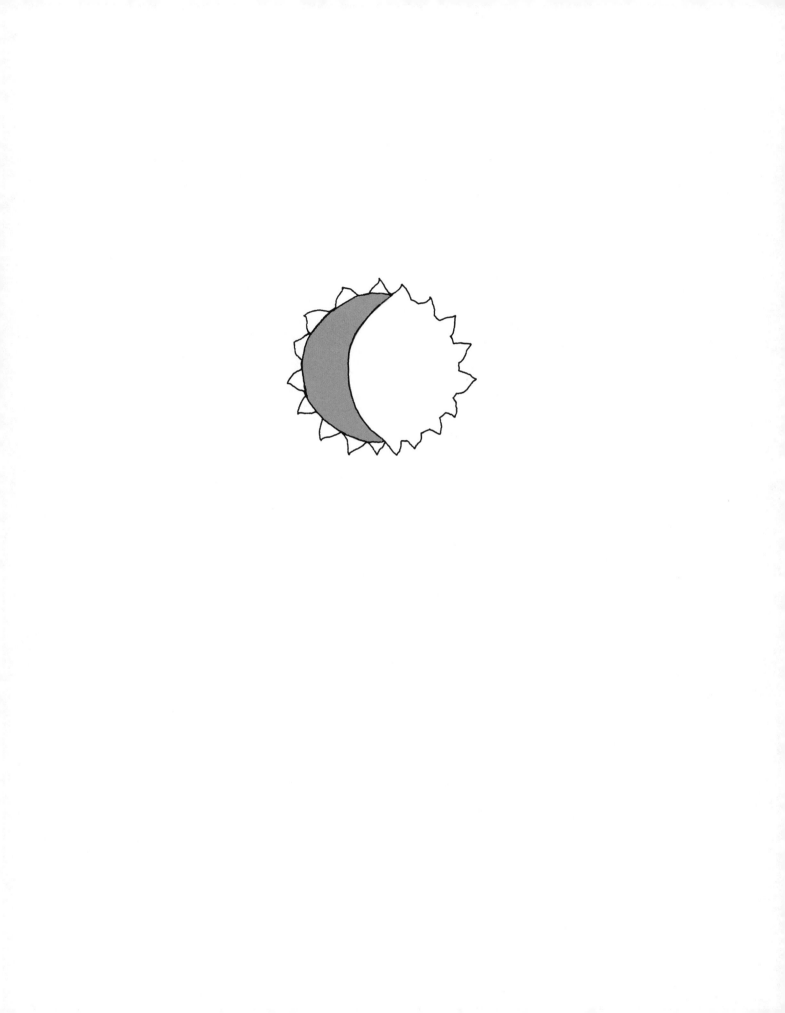

ZONE THERAPY

In Asia for many centuries physicians and healers have been using foot massage as an aid to the diagnosis and treatment of both major and minor health problems. In the West this form of treatment has become known as "zone therapy;" and, more recently, "reflexology." Although largely ignored by the medical profession, it has come to gain a large underground reputation among practitioners of massage.

The principle is simple. For every important organ or muscle area in the trunk and head there is a tiny area that corresponds to it on one or both feet. To locate and treat a health problem affecting any of the upper part of the body you merely massage the corresponding area on the foot.

Sounds crazy? Of course it does to the Western ear — mine as well as yours. But I can only say that I have been experimenting with zone therapy on an informal basis for some time, as have a number of others with whom I am in contact, and I am convinced that there is a great deal to it. It is not a cure-all, and it is definitely no substitute for a visit to the doctor's office. But as a supplement to ordinary medical attention it can often provide a small but noticeable boost in health wherever it is needed.

Why does it work? There are a lot of theories. One frequently advanced is that it is the nervous system which is responsible: numerous nerves running from the foot to elsewhere in the body can cause a reflex action in any other appropriate body part, and this in turn, by stimulating circulation, can bring about a better nutritional intake and elimination of waste in the immediate neighborhood of that same part. Another hypothesis — and my own suspicions are that the truth lies more in this direction — is that the connective tissue and the lymph system throughout the body are the vehicles for energy circuits of a nature as yet unanalyzed by medical science, and that the right kind of massage work on the foot unblocks an energy flow that also effects the corresponding area of the body.

Whatever the reasons, however, zone therapy does seem to work. Here is how you can go about exploring it for yourself.

Arrange yourself and a friend so that the sole of his or her foot is easily accessible to you. If you are working on a massage table I find that the easiest way to do this is to have your friend lying on his back and to seat yourself on a stool so that you are facing the sole of his foot. Another way is to have your friend sit in a chair with one foot propped up on a low padded stool, and either to kneel or to sit on a small cushion facing him.

Next begin massaging the sole of his foot with the tips of your thumbs. Don't bother with oil. Press quite hard; use as much pressure as you would to push a thumbtack into a piece of wood.

And, most essential, press everywhere. Work slowly and thoroughly over the entire sole. Then lift the foot slightly and work the sides of the heel all the way to the ankle bone. What you are looking for are any unusual concentrations of muscular constriction and, more importantly, any reactions of pain on the part of your friend. Stop when you find tightness or when your friend says "Ouch!" Check the accompanying charts, determine what body part corresponds to the right or sore part of the foot, and let your friend know that he has either a health problem or a strong potential for one in that particular part. Then, asking your friend to put up with a little more necessary hurt, continue to massage the same area on the foot with extra care and thoroughness.

Or, if you already know of some health condition that has been bothering your friend, you can go right to the corresponding area of the foot and begin working there.

Frequent short treatments, on the order of ten to twenty minutes once a day or once every two days, are best. Ideally you and your friend should continue with this program both until his condition has improved and until he no longer feels the same sharp soreness as you massage his foot.

A small book on zone therapy worth your investigation: Eunice D. Ingham, *Stories The Feet Can Tell,* printed by Eunice D. Ingham, P.O. Box 948, Rochester, N.Y. 14603. Although next to impossible to find in bookstores, it can be ordered by mail directly from the author.

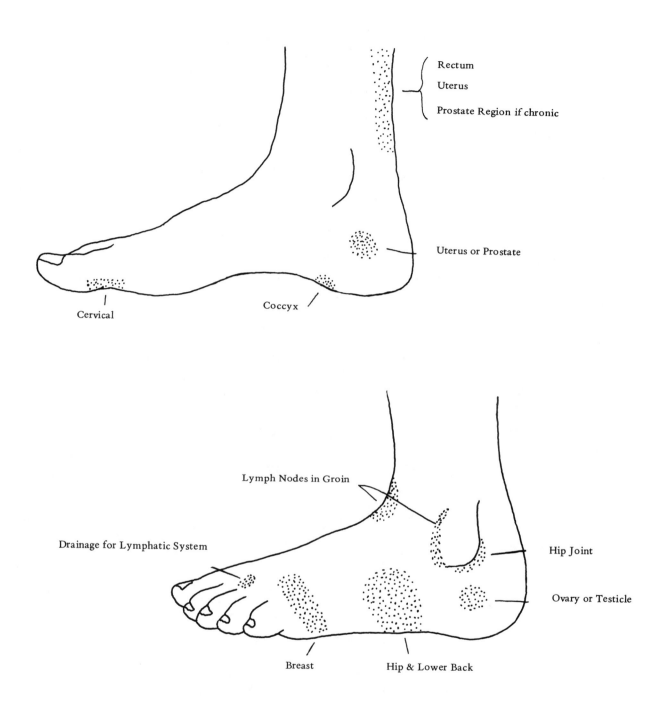

Rectum

Uterus

Prostate Region if chronic

Uterus or Prostate

Cervical

Coccyx

Lymph Nodes in Groin

Drainage for Lymphatic System

Hip Joint

Ovary or Testicle

Breast

Hip & Lower Back

CONNECTIONS ON THE TOP OF BOTH FEET

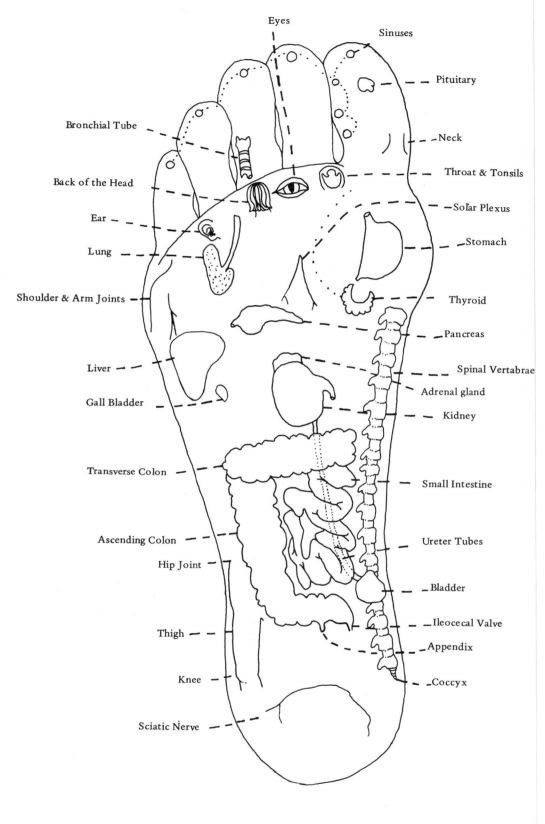

Eyes

Sinuses

Pituitary

Bronchial Tube

Neck

Back of the Head

Throat & Tonsils

Solar Plexus

Ear

Stomach

Lung

Shoulder & Arm Joints

Thyroid

Pancreas

Liver

Spinal Vertabrae

Adrenal gland

Gall Bladder

Kidney

Transverse Colon

Small Intestine

Ascending Colon

Ureter Tubes

Hip Joint

Bladder

Ileocecal Valve

Thigh

Appendix

Knee

Coccyx

Sciatic Nerve

RIGHT FOOT

152

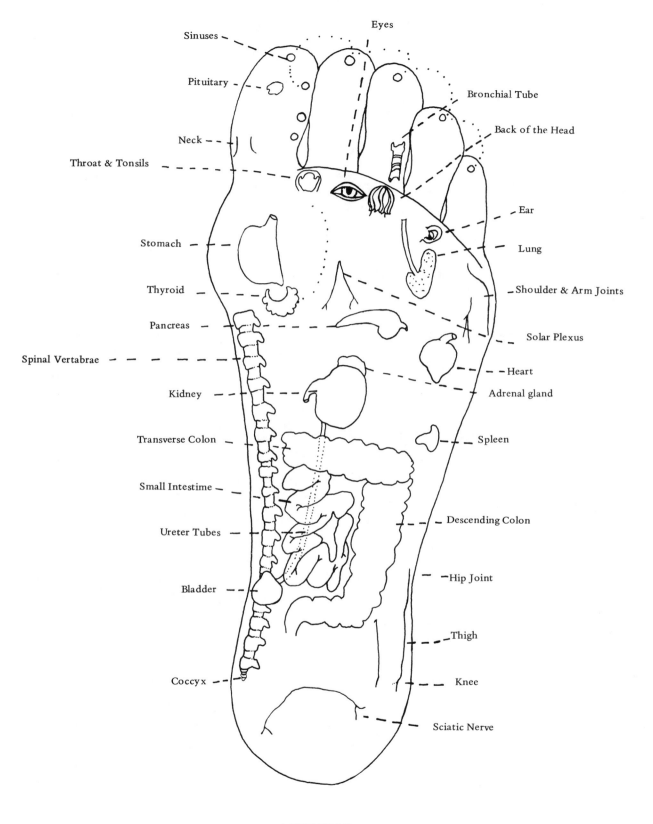

Sinuses

Pituitary

Eyes

Neck

Bronchial Tube

Throat & Tonsils

Back of the Head

Stomach

Ear

Thyroid

Lung

Pancreas

Shoulder & Arm Joints

Spinal Vertabrae

Solar Plexus

Kidney

Heart

Transverse Colon

Adrenal gland

Small Intestime

Spleen

Ureter Tubes

Descending Colon

Bladder

Hip Joint

Thigh

Coccyx

Knee

Sciatic Nerve

LEFT FOOT

OTHER FORMS OF MASSAGE

Once you have begun to make some progress with the type of massage described in this book you will naturally find yourself getting interested in other forms of massage as well. How many other forms actually exist? I've learned from experience not to try to answer this question. Every time I think I know, I find myself suddenly running across two or three totally different massage traditions the likes of which I have never before imagined, let alone heard of.

I want to pass on to you here a series of brief pictures of some of the more prominent among the different approaches to massage that I know. I have already told you about zone therapy. About the others I will limit myself to a more general description, and where I can, will tell you where you can go to find more specific information.

Reichian Massage. Strictly speaking there is no one form of Reichian massage. Wilhelm Reich, a breakaway disciple of Freud now newly famous as the grandfather of what has come to be known as bioenergetic therapy, while working with his patients did apparently use a number of techniques of direct physical contact. Many of these techniques have not only survived, having been handed down by a couple of generations of successors, they have been further extended and developed in several directions by those who have inherited them. What we have today is therefore really a family of related approaches, their two major similarities being their mutual descent from Reich himself and the more or less common goal toward which they are directed.

The chief purpose of Reichian massage — or of whatever we are going to label this general approach — is to assist the dissolution of what Reich called "body armor." Reich found that many individuals subconsciously use muscular constrictedness in various regions of the torso, neck and head as a defense against repressed emotions. By physically working on these areas along with a verbal analysis of the emotions involved, Reich sought to free the body to become a more sensitive and vital receptor of inner feelings.

One of the most common of these methods being used today is an extremely forceful palpitation of key areas of the torso and neck. The amount of massage given any one area varies widely from individual to individual; this must be determined by an analysis of his body and its expressive "blocks." Sharp jabs or pokes designed to stimulate certain reflexes are also sometimes used. So are lighter forms of stroking. In some cases these techniques are also co-ordinated with the cycle of the breath.

This style of massage is rarely practiced by anyone other than a trained therapist. Normally it is made an integral part of a subject's ongoing therapy. Because of its power to release forms of emotional energy that can cause a tremendous immediate anxiety on the part of the subject experiencing them, it should be used only by someone whose professional background equips him to deal with such a therapeutic situation.

Rolfing. Also called Structural Integration, this is a method of deep massage developed over recent decades by Ida Rolf. Its major technique is the application of extremely heavy and concentrated pressure with one knuckle, or an elbow, or sometimes even the knuckles of a fist; often a single point on a subject's body is worked for several seconds at a time. Its purpose is to realign the muscular and connective tissue. Its results are dramatic: a complete reshaping of the body's physical posture.

A Rolfing "treatment" consists ordinarily of ten sessions lasting an hour each. Usually the individual sessions are spaced a week or so apart.

The actual experience of being "Rolfed" is worth mentioning. Usually it is a mixture of strong sensations — extremely painful, yet often exhilirating at the same time. The pain is manageable. It comes only in short bursts of two or three seconds length, and stops immediately when the Rolfer's hand is taken away. It also usually has a curiously solid, almost reassuring quality to it; as opposed, say, to the freakish quality of pain in the dentist's chair. Along with the pain, moreover, often comes an intense and sometimes joyful excitement. One is being physically changed; one can sense muscles cramped for years finally loosening; often energy can be felt moving up and down the entire body.

Other strong emotions are frequently released during the course of the treatment. Sometimes intense childhood memories never before recalled also come to consciousness.

The physical effects of Rolfing are for the most part permanent. A number of subjects have also found that the deep changes in their posture introduced by Rolfing have led to equivalent psychological changes as well. More energy, a greater sense of well-being, and more directness in relating to others are some of the benefits most often cited.

Proskauer massage. A form of direct body treatment developed by Magda Proskauer, a pioneer in what has come to be known as breath therapy. An extremely subtle form of massage, it is closely tied to the rest of her work with the breath. The massage itself is timed to the cycle of the breath; a feather-light touch moving along certain muscle groups during the subject's exhalation is frequently used, for example. Designed to heighten the subject's awareness of and trust in his own breath, when done correctly it leaves one with the sensation of having been massaged from the inside by the breath itself.

Shiatsu. This is a Japanese form of massage done almost entirely within the balls of the thumbs. Of all the Asiatic styles of massage that I know, it is the most easily learned. Pressure is applied with the thumbs for several seconds at a time to any or all of hundreds of points located throughout the body. A complete massage usually covers every part of the body; when done for medical purposes, however, only certain combinations of points may be brought into play.

Shiatsu is tiring to do at first because of the sustained use of the thumbs. Even a tiny bit practiced each day, however, quickly gives the thumbs the necessary strength and endurance.

Besides being an interesting form of massage in its own right, Shiatsu can serve as an extremely effective change of pace when combined with Western forms of massage. It also can be used for self-massage, since many of the points it makes use of can be massaged by a person himself. A good book on the subject, *Shiatsu* by Tokjiru Namikoshi, is available from Japan Publications Trading Company, 1255 Howard St., San Francisco, Calif. 94103.

Acupuncture. A traditional Chinese medical treatment. Based upon an elaborate theory of how energy manifests itself and circulates within the body, acupuncture is done by stimulating key combinations of very precise minute points scattered throughout the body.

As is commonly known, these points are usually stimulated by the insertion of slender metal needles up to a depth of about an inch and a half. Less well known, however, is that acupuncture is also sometimes administered as a form of massage, the necessary points being stimulated by pressure with a knuckle or thumb.

Relatively little of a concrete nature is known about acupuncture in this country, despite its recently having almost overnight become an object of fascination. In the West the most advanced scientific studies of its effects have been made in France, where for some time it has generated excitement within certain medical circles. On the basis of the dramatic and highly sophisticated medical cures acupuncture is reported consistently to achieve, one can't help but hope that a more sustained program of research may someday bring about a sweeping transformation of our scientific understanding of the human body.

Polarity Therapy. This is the name given by Dr. Randolph Stone to his own comprehensive integration of a number of massage and manipulation techniques which he has developed over the course of half a century.

Perhaps the easiest way to describe polarity therapy is that it looks like Rolfing and thinks like acupuncture. Like Rolfing, it makes frequent use of heavy concentrated pressure applied with a knuckle, thumb or elbow. Again like Rolfing, one of its functions is to bring about a realignment of the posture of the body.

Like acupuncture, however, the practice of polarity therapy rests upon an extremely detailed analysis of the nature of energy flow within the body. Much of this theory is derived from yogic and spiritual traditions in India. Dr. Stone himself, a lifelong student of meditation, has spent many years in India, and is the director of a medical clinic there.

A list of Dr. Stone's publications is available upon request from 7557 S. Merrill Ave., Chicago 49, Illinois.

WHERE TO LEARN MORE

Once you have mastered the strokes in this book, how can you widen your knowledge of massage technique?

One of the best ways is to find friends who are also into massage, and, like travelling folksingers and other craftsmen, to trade what you know for what they know. This may not look like a viable option — fellow massage connaisseurs may not seem to be on the horizon at the moment — but I assure you that the laws of the universe are such that it is impossible to know and love massage and not sooner or later to run into others who feel the same way. You'll see.

Another excellent place to go, is to a good workshop in massage at a growth center such as Esalen Institute. With an instructor at a workshop you can check out how you are doing with what you have already learned, and can pick up many new strokes and techniques as well. More important, you will receive a more thorough grounding in massage as a means of communication, trust, and freeing blocked energy. A list of over a hundred growth centers throughout the country is available from the Association of Humanist Psychology, 548 Page St., San Francisco 94117. Lists of growth centers are also to be found in the closing pages of Jane Howard's *Please Touch: A Guided Tour of the Human Potential Movement* (New York: McGraw-Hill, 1970), and also of Howard R. Lewis and Harold S. Stretfeld's *Growth Games* (New York: Harcourt Brace, 1970).

Esalen itself conducts workshops in both San Francisco and Big Sur, California. For further information write Esalen Institute, 1776 Union St., San Francisco, Calif. 94123.

Free universities occasionally offer courses in massage. I have known of several that were quite good.

Formal schools of massage are to be found in some large cities. Most offer a single course lasting anywhere from six weeks to six months. Their emphasis tends to be almost entirely upon the technical side of massage. A small amount of anatomy is often taught as well. Check out a school thoroughly before applying, as they vary greatly in quality.

Finally, you have your hands, your best teachers. Keep listening.

THE PROFESSIONAL WORLDS OF MASSAGE

Perhaps by this time massage has come to interest you enough that the idea of doing it on a professional basis looks appealing. If so, what I have to say can, I'm afraid, only discourage you.

In this country there are at least three distinct professional worlds of massage. They are very different from one another, and there is no getting around the fact that there exists little communication or understanding among them.

The world of massage most prominent in the public eye is that of the professional massage studio. Largely confined to big cities, their public image is about on a par with that of the dime-a-dance halls of a generation ago.

This notorious reputation is only partially deserved. In point of fact the studios vary widely among themselves. A few (in most cities a very small number, if any at all) are actually fronts for prostitution. Many others, although in fact offering strictly legitimate massage, seek by means of lurid advertising to capitalize upon this image. Unfortunately, even though their customers learn quickly enough what is and what isn't on the menu, this style of promotion serves only to reinforce in the public mind the same bastardized image of massage.

The atmosphere of most legitimate studios is at worst shabby, at best clinical. Although there exist some wonderful exceptions, the massage offered is usually of a strikingly low quality. In many cases the masseuses have received only a minimal amount of training, if any. In other cases they are more than competent, but tend to react to the tedium and the unpleasant vibrations in their working situation by giving an impersonal and mechanical massage.

Needless to say, I cannot recommend your looking for a job in a studio with much enthusiasm. As someone who enjoys doing massage (I assume this is one reason you would like to make it your work), you stand to be continually frustrated; the average client, thanks to the advertising he has been exposed to, will bring with him so many expectations along other lines that he will have a difficult time listening to what your hands really have to say. And as a woman (massage studios almost never employ men), or so I am told, you will find yourself repeatedly cast in an unpleasant and stereotyped role.

Going to other people's homes to do massage — doing "outcalls," as it is called in the trade — is really an extension of the studio scene and presents most of the same difficulties. In many states a local business liscense, usually available immediately upon payment of a small fee, is all that is legally required to do outcalls. Practically what it means is investing in a portable massage table (see the previous chapter on tables); arranging for transportation (a car is almost always necessary); advertising, either informally through friends and acquaintances or, as is usually necessary, through a local newspaper; and then waiting by the phone.

The advantages of doing outcalls are that you are your own boss, that you can usually expect to be paid more for the actual amount of time that you spend doing massage, and that over the course of time it can sometimes be a little easier to collect a regular clientele of the type with which you wish to work. For the most part, however, you will be subject to the same psychological unpleasantness that you would encounter in a studio, since here as elsewhere the distorted public image of massage acts as a kind of filter selecting who will call you and what his expectations are likely to be.

Men can do outcalls as well as women. Most find themselves subject to many of the same hassles.

A quite different type of massage scene is to be found in the physical therapy room of most hospitals. Here massage is performed by trained physical therapists for strictly medical purposes. For the right person with the right credentials this can be a reasonable professional outlet for massage. For many, however, it suffers from several limitations.

First, you must be licensed as a physical therapist. In most states this means at least a year of full-time formal schooling leading to a degree in physical therapy. Second, as a physical therapist massage will be only a part of what you will be expected to do; and when massage is prescribed, it will usually be only for extensive work on a single part of the body. Third, although free from the sexual ambiguities of the massage studio, the atmosphere of the hospital tends to be equally impersonal.

Some gymnasiums and health clubs also have massage rooms. Their atmosphere tends to be more like that of the hospital than anything else. No formal degree is ordinarily required.

Yet another world of massage is that of the growth movement. As I have already said, there are a number of growth centers, such as Esalen, where one can learn massage. A smaller number also have one or several masseurs or masseuses on hand in order to make massage available to members of workshops.

Comparitively speaking, those who hold such jobs tend to find them quite satisfying. One reason is that most of the people who come for workshops at a growth center tune in quite easily to the value and meaning of massage. Another reason is that the atmosphere of a growth center, where yoga, Tai Chi, and other forms of "body work" are also frequently taught, is often a stimulating one. Yet it is precisely these advantages, coupled with the tiny number of positions available, that make these jobs next to impossible to find. By all means try if you want; and good luck. But be prepared to be disappointed.

If, despite all this discouraging advice, you are still convinced that you want to do massage professionally, I do have one suggestion of a more positive nature: if you can't find the scene you want, then make your own. If the growth movement whets your appetite, for example, then find a growth center that *doesn't* have a massage room and persuade them that they need one and need you to run it.

Or, if working in a studio appeals to you, start a small one of your own. Make the atmosphere as pleasant as you yourself would like it to be, keep your advertising tasteful, and put in a little effort to teaching those who come to you what massage is all about. Here in the Bay Area I have already seen one friend make this formula work beautifully. It can be done!

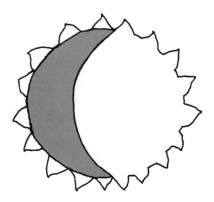

ANATOMY

The more I teach massage, the more convinced I become that anyone learning massage for the first time is best off *not* studying formal anatomy until he has mastered some of the basic massage techniques. The reason for this is simple. In the beginning what you need to learn above all else is the art of tuning in with your hands, of being able to "read," through the sense of touch alone, the overall feel and architecture of another person's body. Learning formal anatomy right from the start tends, I feel, to detract from rather than hasten the development of this sensitivity. Moreover, as I have stressed several times earlier, a knowledge of anatomy is in no way necessary for the learning of most basic techniques themselves.

Why then bother to study anatomy at all? For several very good reasons. Most important is that it will give you extra confidence. And, as I have mentioned, a knowledge of anatomy will help you to develop new massage techniques from those you have already learned. Also it can be of considerable help when dealing with certain problems — extreme tension concentrated in a particular muscular area, for example. Finally, it will satisfy some of your curiosity about how the human body really functions — and believe me, if you do a lot of massage, this is a subject that sooner or later will begin to fascinate you.

The following remarks and diagrams are designed merely to provide you with a brief overview. For more extensive discussions of anatomy see the bibliography in "Some More Reading."

The skeleton. The bones themselves making up the skeleton have no "feeling." However, the nerve sheaths which encase them do, as does the connective tissue which attaches muscles to the bones. The bones also have important chemical and structural functions in the body. For massage, however, their main interest is their ability to serve as landmarks for muscle groups and areas of nerve sensation.

The long bones are always curved. These curves increase the elasticity of the bones, provide more attachment surface for muscles, and give special direction to certain portions of muscle.

There are approximately 206 separate bones in the human body. Make yourself familiar with some of the more important ones and you will be able to find your way around anywhere on the body.

The skull. The skull rests on top of the spine, directly upon the topmost spinal vertabra which is called the Atlas. The skull is made up of many smaller bones, including the cranium, which covers the brain, and the bones of the face. These bones are fused, however; for practical purposes you can consider them one piece, with the exception of the jaw.

The spine consists of 24 separate vertabrae extending from the base of the skull to the base of the lumbar region, plus the sacrum and the coccyx.

There are 7 vertabrae in the neck (cervical vertabrae); 12 vertabrae in the upper portion of the back (dorsal), to which are attached the ribs; and 5 vertabrae in the lower back (lumbar). The sacrum and the coccyx consist at birth of separate and moveable vertabrae; however, over the course of time these vertabrae slowly fuse together until, usually by the time their owner has reached 30 years of age, they have become one immoveable bone. In general, up and down the entire spine, the lower the vertabrae the bigger in all dimensions it will be.

Each of those bumps which you can see along the spine is actually what is called a "process," a spiny protective point sticking out of the main portion of the vertabra itself. With slight variations each vertabra is shaped like the illustration below, having a cylindrical base with an enclosure behind for the spinal cord, and three boney processes, pointing to each side and directly backwards. If you press with your fingers you can usually feel all three processes.

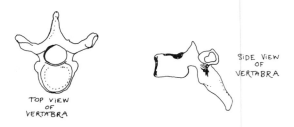

TOP VIEW OF VERTABRA

SIDE VIEW OF VERTABRA

Between the cylindrical sections of each pair of vertabrae rests a cartilage disc which cushions the vertabra during movement. Occasionally one of these discs can give a little to one side — the notorious "slipped disc."

The normal curve of the human spine is like so:

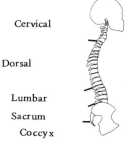

Cervical

Dorsal

Lumbar
Sacrum
Coccyx

The sternum is the hard flat ridge in the center of the chest to which the ribs are attached in front.

The clavicles are the two narrow protruding bones at the very top of the chest. They extend from the top of the sternum to the shoulders.

The ribs, usually twelve in number, form the thorax and attach in back to the twelve thoracic vertabrae. In front, the top seven ribs are attached directly to the sternum. The next three are attached to the sternum indirectly by bands of cartilage so hard that they in turn feel like bone to the touch. The last two are called floating ribs because they attach only to the vertebrae in back. The bottom-most floating rib can present many surprises when you look for it with your fingers. Often you will find it in the "right" position as shown in the diagram; sometimes, however, it slants downward at a much sharper angle, in which case its lower tip is likely to show up buried in the muscles of the torso at a point not much higher than the hip.

The scapulae, or shoulder blades, are a particularly curious pair of bones from the point of view of massage. The first interesting item is their shape; note especially the acromian process, a sort of penisula reaching up and to the side to connect with the clavicle at the shoulder. Note also the structural role which the scapula plays at the shoulder; the scapula and the clavicle alone form the entire architectural setting for the socket into which the humerus, the thick bone of the upper arm, is fitted. Finally, the clavicle is the *only* other bone to which the scapula is attached; although lying "against" the ribs in back (some muscle and connective tissue actually lies between them), it is free to move over them an inch or more in every direction.

The arm. Notice that the upper arm consists of one bone whereas the forearm consists of two.

The hand consists of many tiny bones. The wrist alone contains eight.

The pelvis. The main thing about the pelvic girdle is that for all practical purposes it consists of one large basin-shaped bone. Each large hip bone consists originally of three bones which with maturation become fused, and both hip bones in turn become so tightly connected to the sacrum that the entire structure feels to the fingers like a single bone.

The greatest difference between the male and female skelton is to be found in the pelvis. The female pelvic bones are wider apart, and also lighter and shorter. The male pelvic bones are broader, and have larger processes and ridges.

Because the pelvic structure is one large bone, movement of this area is achieved only by bending either the thigh joints or the spine itself where it meets the sacrum at the fifth lumbar vertabra. The immediate area surrounding the fifth lumbar is for this reason a foremost candidate for some good massage work on almost everyone.

The leg, like the arm, consists mainly of one large bone on top and two parallel bones below. The patella, or kneecap, is a small shield of bone buried in a large tendon and is not attached directly to any other bone. At the top of the femur, the huge bone of the thigh, note the greater trocanter sticking to the side. An important point of orientation for the observer, the visible bump produced by the greater trocanter is often mistakely thought to be a part of the hip.

The foot, like the hand, is an intricate arrangement of numerous small bones.

The muscles, the intricate webbing of the body, are more than two hundred in number. They vary greatly in both size and shape. Some are smaller than your fingernail, others a good deal wider and longer than your entire hand. Some are cord-like, others are thick masses, and still others are flat sheets.

Surrounding each muscle is a fibrous sheath called connective tissue or fascia. Several layers of connective tissue also lie between the entire muscular system and the skin itself. The deepest layer of connective tissue actually constitutes a single continuous matrix, enclosing and even permeating the internal structure of each individual muscle.

Most muscles are attached in two or more places to two or more different bones; some, however, are attached at one or more points to the connective tissue adjoining other muscles. Movement in the body is made possible by entire groups of muscles working in unison, some relaxing at the same time that others contract.

In addition to studying the accompanying diagrams (drawn after Albinus) you might profitably spend some time with one or more good anatomical texts with pictures of individual muscles and muscle groups. I have included several in the bibliography in "Some More Reading."

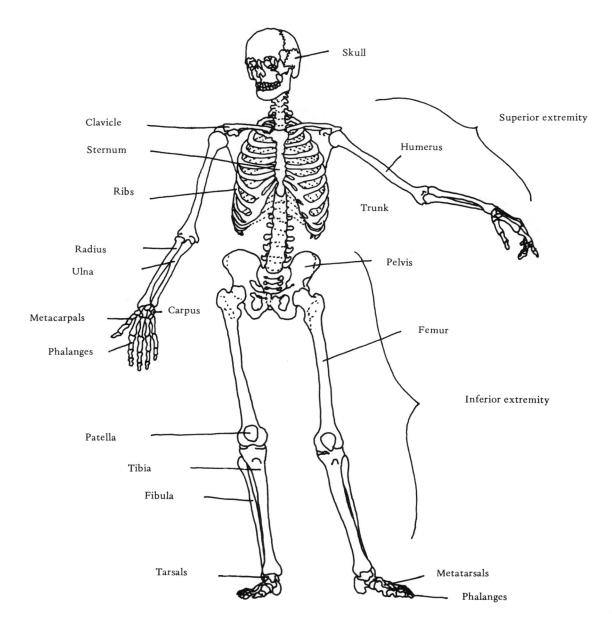

Skull

Clavicle

Sternum

Ribs

Radius

Ulna

Metacarpals

Carpus

Phalanges

Superior extremity

Humerus

Trunk

Pelvis

Femur

Inferior extremity

Patella

Tibia

Fibula

Tarsals

Metatarsals

Phalanges

SKELETON, FRONT VIEW

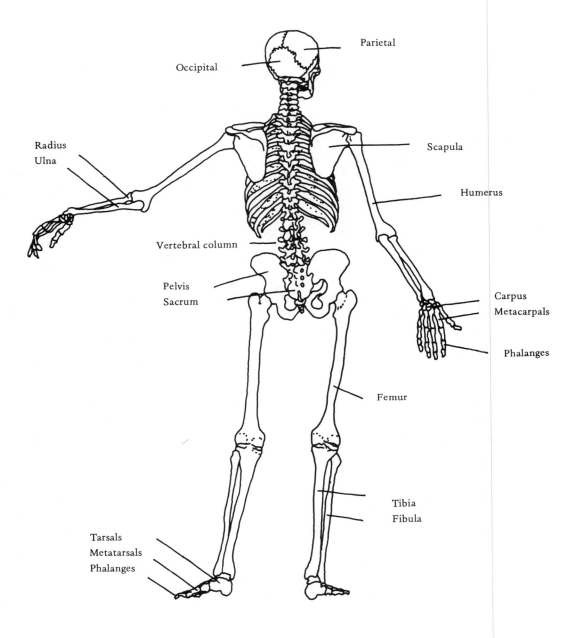

Parietal

Occipital

Radius
Ulna

Scapula

Humerus

Vertebral column

Carpus
Metacarpals

Pelvis
Sacrum

Phalanges

Femur

Tibia
Fibula

Tarsals
Metatarsals
Phalanges

SKELETON, BACK VIEW

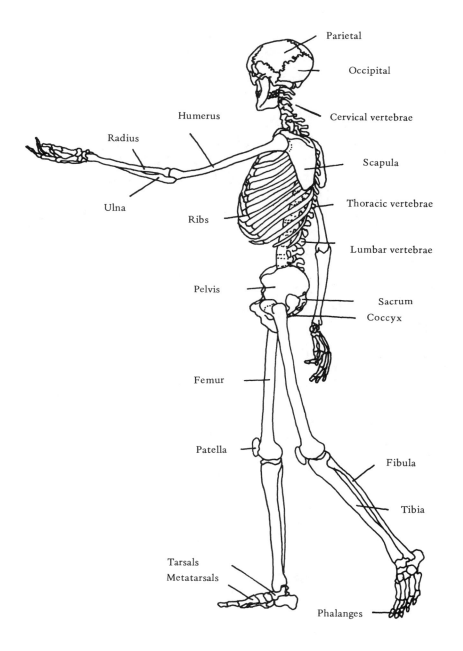

Parietal

Occipital

Cervical vertebrae

Humerus

Radius

Scapula

Ulna

Thoracic vertebrae

Ribs

Lumbar vertebrae

Pelvis

Sacrum

Coccyx

Femur

Patella

Fibula

Tibia

Tarsals
Metatarsals

Phalanges

SKELETON, SIDE VIEW

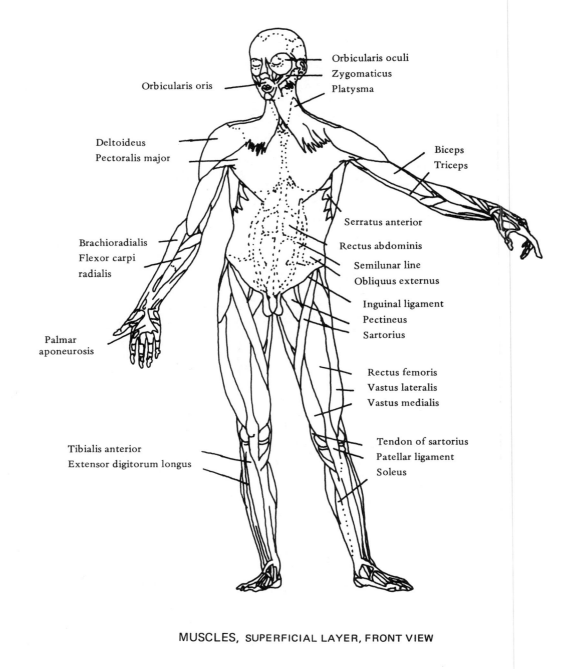

Orbicularis oculi
Zygomaticus
Platysma

Orbicularis oris

Deltoideus
Pectoralis major

Biceps
Triceps

Serratus anterior

Rectus abdominis

Brachioradialis
Flexor carpi
radialis

Semilunar line
Obliquus externus

Inguinal ligament
Pectineus
Sartorius

Palmar
aponeurosis

Rectus femoris
Vastus lateralis
Vastus medialis

Tibialis anterior
Extensor digitorum longus

Tendon of sartorius
Patellar ligament
Soleus

MUSCLES, SUPERFICIAL LAYER, FRONT VIEW

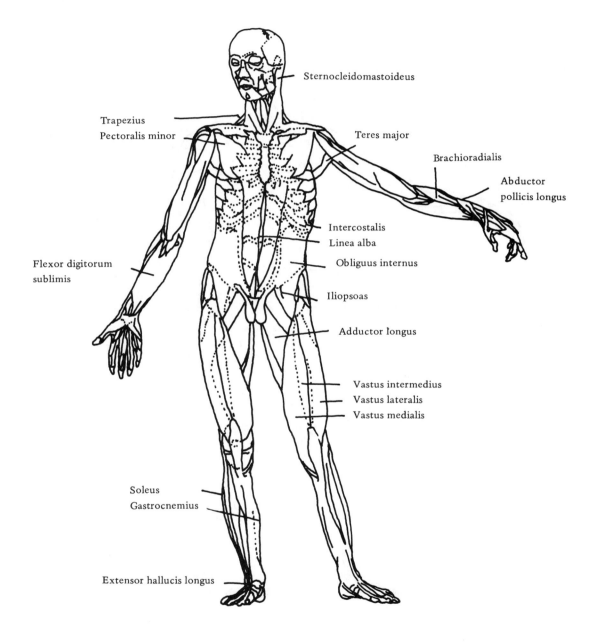

Sternocleidomastoideus

Trapezius

Pectoralis minor

Teres major

Brachioradialis

Abductor
pollicis longus

Intercostalis

Linea alba

Obliguus internus

Flexor digitorum
sublimis

Iliopsoas

Adductor longus

Vastus intermedius

Vastus lateralis

Vastus medialis

Soleus

Gastrocnemius

Extensor hallucis longus

MUSCLES, DEEP LAYER, FRONT VIEW

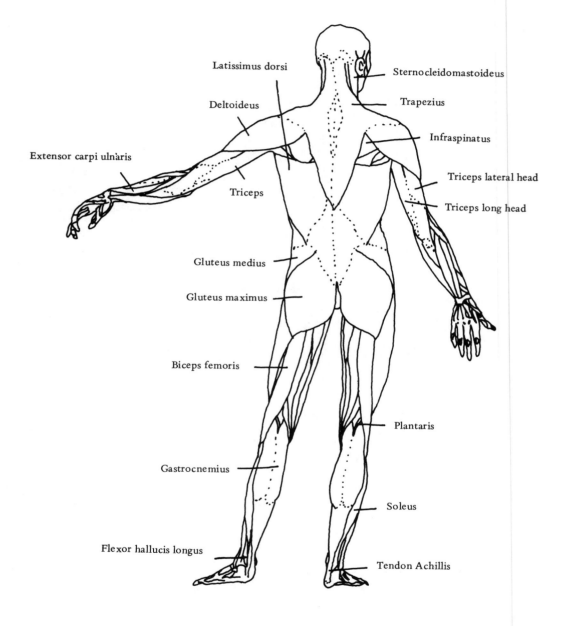

Latissimus dorsi

Deltoideus

Extensor carpi ulnàris

Triceps

Sternocleidomastoideus

Trapezius

Infraspinatus

Triceps lateral head

Triceps long head

Gluteus medius

Gluteus maximus

Biceps femoris

Plantaris

Gastrocnemius

Soleus

Flexor hallucis longus

Tendon Achillis

MUSCLES, SUPERFICIAL LAYER, BACK VIEW

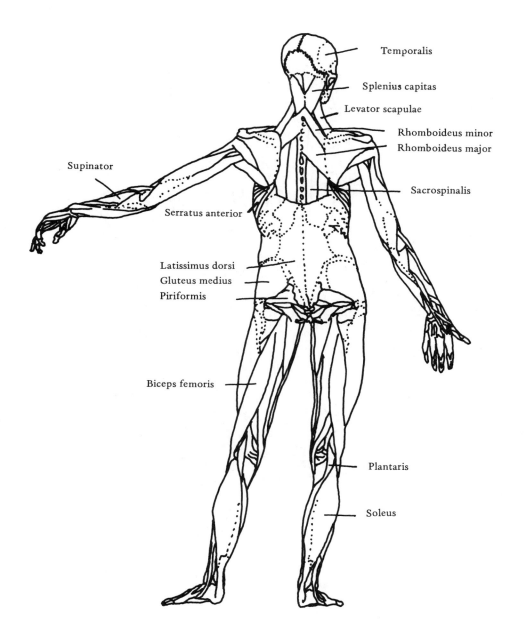

Temporalis

Splenius capitas

Levator scapulae

Rhomboideus minor
Rhomboideus major

Sacrospinalis

Supinator

Serratus anterior

Latissimus dorsi
Gluteus medius
Piriformis

Biceps femoris

Plantaris

Soleus

MUSCLES, DEEP LAYER, BACK VIEW

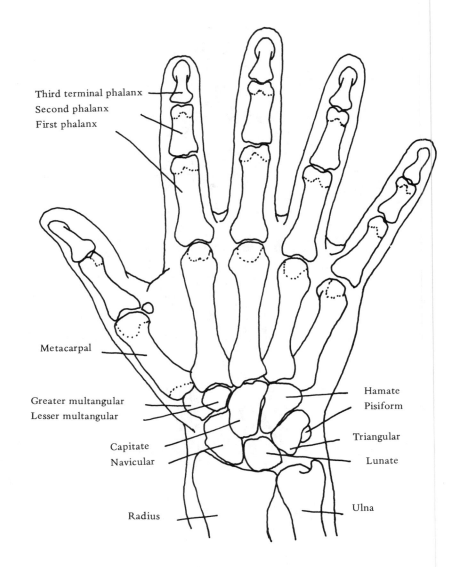

Third terminal phalanx
Second phalanx
First phalanx

Metacarpal

Greater multangular
Lesser multangular

Capitate
Navicular

Radius

Hamate
Pisiform

Triangular

Lunate

Ulna

BONES OF THE HAND, RIGHT PALM VIEW

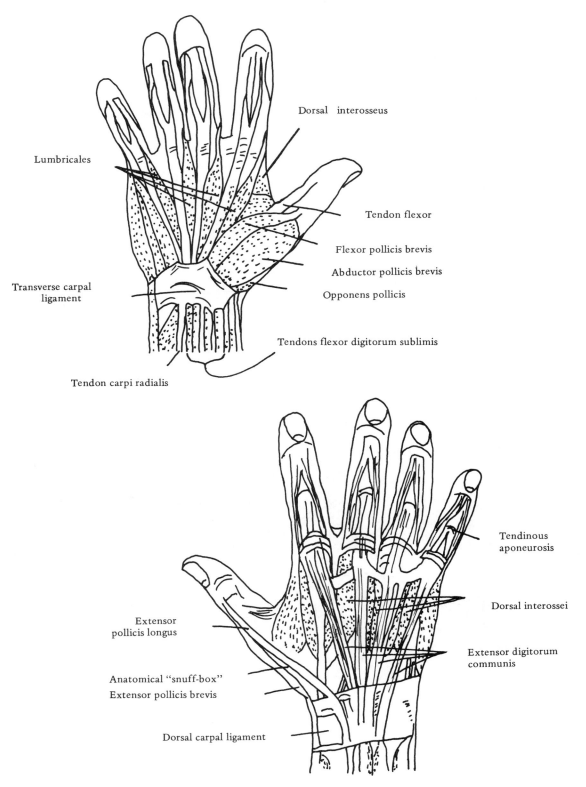

Dorsal interosseus

Lumbricales

Tendon flexor

Flexor pollicis brevis

Abductor pollicis brevis

Transverse carpal
ligament

Opponens pollicis

Tendons flexor digitorum sublimis

Tendon carpi radialis

Extensor
pollicis longus

Tendinous
aponeurosis

Dorsal interossei

Anatomical "snuff-box"
Extensor pollicis brevis

Extensor digitorum
communis

Dorsal carpal ligament

MUSCLES OF THE HAND, TOP VIEW

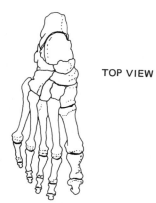

TOP VIEW

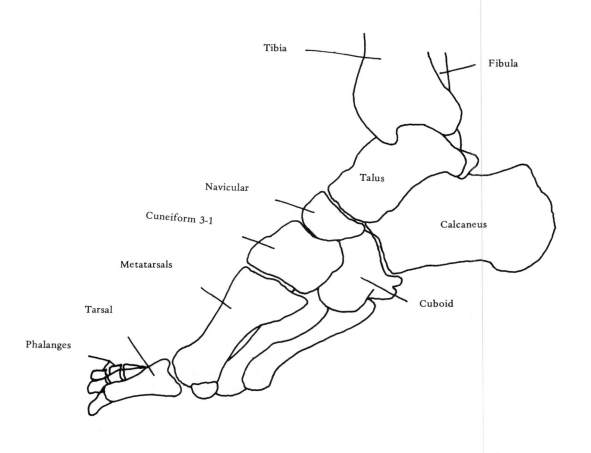

Tibia

Fibula

Talus

Navicular

Cuneiform 3-1

Calcaneus

Metatarsals

Tarsal

Cuboid

Phalanges

BONES OF THE FOOT, RIGHT INSIDE VIEW

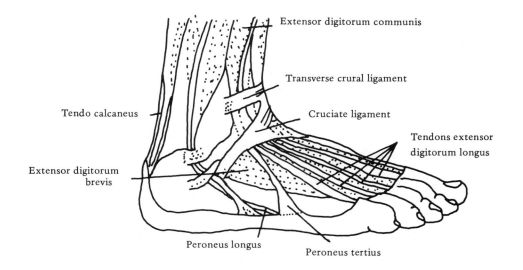

Extensor digitorum communis

Transverse crural ligament

Cruciate ligament

Tendo calcaneus

Tendons extensor digitorum longus

Extensor digitorum brevis

Peroneus longus

Peroneus tertius

MUSCLES OF THE FOOT, OUTER VIEW

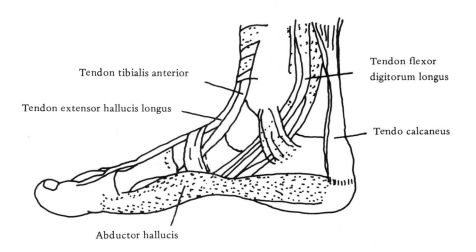

Tendon tibialis anterior

Tendon flexor digitorum longus

Tendon extensor hallucis longus

Tendo calcaneus

Abductor hallucis

MUSCLES OF THE FOOT, INNER VIEW

SOME READING

About massage itself there is not much more to read. Older books on massage tend to be funky but extremely short on practical information. Of more interest, and still available in print, are the following:

Gertrude Beard and Elizabeth C. Wood, *Massage: Principles and Techniques,* W.B. Saunders.

Bernard Gunther, *What To Do Until The Messiah Comes,* Collier.

Eunice D. Ingham, *Stories The Feet Can Tell,* printed by Eunice D. Ingham, Post Office Box 948, Rochester, N.Y. 14603.

Tokujiro Namikoshi, *Shiatsu,* Japan Publications.

Some decent inexpensive books on anatomy:

Edmond J. Farris, *Art Students' Anatomy,* Dover.

Walter T. Foster, *Anatomy,* Foster Art Service.

Clem W. Thompson, *Manual Of Structural Kinesiology.*

The most thorough standard reference work on anatomy:

Gray, Henry, *Anatomy of the Human Body,* ed. 27. (edited by Charles Mayo Goss), 1959, Lea & Febiger.

A difficult but important philosphic account of the relation between mind and body:

Maurice Merleau-Ponty, *The Phenomenology Of Perception,* Routledge & Kegan Paul.

On the importance of the body in psychology:

Stanley Keleman, *Sexuality, Self, & Survival,* Lodestar Press.

Alexander Lowen, *The Betrayal Of The Body,* Collier.

Wilhelm Reich, *Character Analysis,* Noonday.

Wilhelm Reich, *The Function Of The Orgasm,* Noonday.

William C. Schutz, *Here Comes Everybody,* Harper & Row.

Several overviews of the human potential movement:
Jane Howard, *Please Touch: A Guided Tour Of The Human Potential Movement*, McGraw.
Severin Peterson, *A Catalog Of The Ways People Grow*, Ballantine.

On gestalt therapy:
Frederick Perls, Ralph F. Hefferline, Paul Goodman, *Gestalt Therapy*, Delta.
Frederick Perls, *Gestalt Therapy Verbatim*, Real People Press.

On techniques you can use at home to get more acquainted with yourself and your body:
Bernard Gunther, *Sense Relaxation Below Your Mind*, Collier.
Howard R. Lewis and Dr. Harold S. Streitfeld, *Growth Games: How To Tune In Yourself, Your Family, Your Friends*, Harcourt Brace, Jovanovich.

On meditation:
Christmas Humphreys, *Concentration And Meditation*, Shambala.
Philip Kapleau, ed., *Three Pillars Of Zen*, Beacon.
Claudio Naranjo and Robert E. Ornstein, *On The Psychology Of Meditation*, Viking.
Shunryu Suzuki, *Zen Mind, Beginner's Mind*, Weatherhill.

On yoga:
B.K.S. Iyengar, *Light On Yoga*, Schocken.
Yogiraj Sri Swami Satchidananda, *Integral Yoga Hatha*, Holt, Rinehard & Winston.

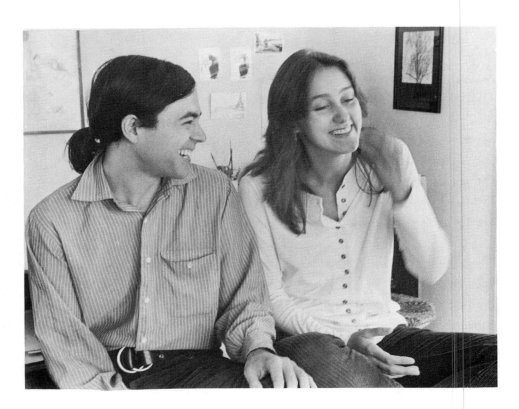

ABOUT THE AUTHOR, THE ILLUSTRATOR, AND HOW THIS BOOK WAS MADE

George Downing

The Bay Area has been my home for some years now. I'm a member of the teaching staff of Esalen Institute in San Francisco, and I lead workshops and classes for Esalen and other growth centers in massage and in body awareness. I myself learned massage from Storm Accioli, Molly Day Schackman, other teachers and numerous friends. My most helpful teacher in the human potential movement has been Magda Proskauer, with whom I have studied the techniques of breath therapy for some time. Kent and I frequently lead workshops together.

Anne Kent Rush

I've lived in many parts of the United States. Now the Bay Area is my home.

In the country in Maryland when I was small I drew the things around me. I've kept drawing in spite of most schools and because of a few teachers and friends.

For several years I have been doing commercial art work, mainly book illustration and covers. Books to me are messages to be received as a whole — type and shapes and spaces and feeling. I also do a great deal of yoga, Tai Chi Chuan and massage, and lead workshops in massage and body awareness. Polarity therapy is currently my main work.

The Book

It all started when Kent and I began looking for a good book on massage, something which we could recommend both to those who had already learned massage from us and to those who had never had any formal instruction at all. Few books proved to be available; none looked satisfactory. Since writing is something I have always enjoyed and since Kent when she is not leading groups is a free-lance book designer, the next step was a natural one: we decided to create our own book.

We broke ground by writing an introductory chapter, writing and illustrating a few representative strokes from what would later become the instruction section, and making a tentative outline of the other chapters in the book. We chose to take what we had gotten on paper to The Bookworks, a publishing firm in Berkeley for whom Kent had already done some art work; we knew that The Bookworks was trying to set a new direction in the publishing world by letting authors have a larger say about the physical appearance of their books, and this greatly appealed to us. Don Gerrard, editor of The Bookworks, liked what we showed him. At that time The Bookworks had just entered into an agreement with Random House in New York whereby the two firms would jointly publish certain books; Don proposed that our book be published so. We agreed, and signed a joint contract with both firms. Then, for months to follow, to work!

Work it was. Much of it we loved, much was utter frustration. The decisions were endless. Photographs or drawings? Line drawings, we decided by experiment, both felt less slick and "read" more easily in relation to the text. Hardbound or paper? An edition in paper, we decided, would immediately make the book available to many more people. Then there were questions of the particular shade of paper and ink, of the style of type, of margins and paragraph spacing and a hundred smaller items. We chose cream paper and brown ink; they felt warm to us. We picked out 12 point Aldine Roman, a type that looked large and readable, and decided to have a little extra space between the lines and to have the instruction section set in bold face so that the book could be easily read while lying open next to someone actually trying out some massage. We even tried to figure out a way to prevent the pages from being stained by oil spots. No luck. Watch your oil bottle.

Numerous friends were of great help. Some spent long hours with us posing for the photographs from which Kent made most of the drawings; many others took sections of the book, tested them, and gave us much invaluable feedback. Jim Howland helped proofread every page. Dorothy Pitts and Vera Allen of Hayward, the typesetters of this book, were endlessly resourceful when presented with the special problem of setting the type around the drawings in the manner which we wanted. Above all Don, our editor, helped us every inch of the way with his advice, encouragement and friendship.

Finally the end came, the book looked as finished as it was ever going to be, and we let Don mail it off to New York and then settled ourselves down for the intervening wait — the additional months that it takes for a book to be printed, shipped to a warehouse, publicized, ordered, and mailed to bookstores. Now its yours.

We would enjoy hearing how you like this book and of what use and meaning it has been to you. Write us c/o Random House, 201 East 50th Street, New York, New York 10022.

Also available from Random House/Bookworks:
Edited by Don Gerrard

394-73113-1   **SEEING WITH THE MIND'S EYE,** Samuels & Samuels, M.D. (paper)

394-58769-3   **THE WELL CAT BOOK,** McGinnis, D.V.M. (cloth)

394-58768-5   **THE WELL DOG BOOK,** McGinnis, D.V.M. (cloth)